3/04 ✓2015

D0225372

DATING AND SEXUALITY IN AMERICA

A Reference Handbook

Other Titles in ABC-CLIO's
CONTEMPORARY WORLD ISSUES
Series

Books in the Contemporary World Issues series address vital issues in today's society such as genetic engineering, pollution, and biodiversity. Written by professional writers, scholars, and nonacademic experts, these books are authoritative, clearly written, up-to-date, and objective. They provide a good starting point for research by high school and college students, scholars, and general readers as well as by legislators, businesspeople, activists, and others.

Each book, carefully organized and easy to use, contains an overview of the subject, a detailed chronology, biographical sketches, facts and data and/or documents and other primary-source material, a directory of organizations and agencies, annotated lists of print and nonprint resources, and an index.

Readers of books in the Contemporary World Issues series will find the information they need in order to have a better understanding of the social, political, environmental, and economic issues facing the world today.

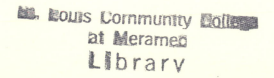

DATING AND SEXUALITY IN AMERICA

A Reference Handbook

Jeffrey S. Turner

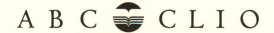

A B C CLIO

Santa Barbara, California • Denver, Colorado • Oxford, England

Library of Congress Cataloging-in-Publication Data

Turner, Jeffrey S.
Dating and sexuality in America : a reference handbook / Jeffrey S.
Turner.
    p. cm. — (Contemporary world issues)
Includes bibliographical references and index.
    ISBN 1-85109-584-5 (hardcover : alk. paper); 1-85109-589-6 (eBook)
    1. Dating (Social customs)—United States. 2. Teenagers—United
States—Social life and customs. 3. Teenagers—United States—Conduct
of life. 4. Teenagers—Sexual behavior. 5. Dating (Social
customs)—Cross-cultural studies. I. Title. II. Series.
    HQ801.A3T87 2003
    306.73'0973—dc22
    2003014917   1851095845

07 06 05 04 03   10 9 8 7 6 5 4 3 2 1

This book is also available on the World Wide Web as an eBook.
Visit abc-clio.com for details.

ABC-CLIO, Inc.
130 Cremona Drive, P.O. Box 1911
Santa Barbara, California 93116-1911

This book is printed on acid-free paper ∞.
Manufactured in the United States of America

Dedicated to Carla Roberts

Contents

Preface, xiii
Acknowledgements, xiv

1 Background and History, 1
The Early 1900s, 4
The "Roaring Twenties," 8
World War II, 10
The Sexual Revolution, 13
The Twenty-First Century, 17
Summary, 20
References, 21

2 Issues, Controversies, and Solutions, 25
Dating and Sexual Values, 27
Media Impact on Dating and Sexuality, 31
Internet Romance and Sex, 36
Dating and Club Drugs, 40
Date Rape, 45
Same-Sex Dating, 49
Premarital Sex, 52
Birth Control, 55
Teenage Pregnancy, 58
Sexually Transmitted Diseases, 61
Living Together, 64
Teenage Marriages, 66
Dating and Sexuality Education, 69
Summary, 73
References, 76

3 Worldwide Perspective, 85
Australia, 86
China, 88
France, 90
India, 92

Indonesia, 93
Ireland, 95
Japan, 97
Latin America and the Caribbean, 98
The Middle East and North Africa, 100
The Russian Federation, 102
Sub-Saharan Africa, 104
Sweden, 106
United Kingdom, 108
Summary, 110
References, 112

4 Chronology, 115

5 Biographical Sketches, 129
Bordo, Susan R., 129
Brooks-Gunn, Jeanne, 130
Calderone, Mary S., 131
Cherlin, Andrew J., 132
Coles, Robert, 132
DeLamater, John D., 133
Donnerstein, Edward, 134
Elias, Maurice J., 134
Erikson, Erik H., 135
Freud, Sigmund, 136
Fromm, Erich, 137
Furstenberg, Frank F., Jr., 138
Galinsky, Ellen, 138
Gelles, Richard J., 139
Gilligan, Carol, 140
Gordon, Sol, 141
Haffner, Debra W., 142
Hetherington, E. Mavis, 143
Hyde, Janet S., 144
Kinsey, Alfred C., 144
Kohlberg, Lawrence, 145
Maccoby, Eleanor E., 146
Maslow, Abraham H., 147
Masters, William H. and Johnson, Virginia A., 148
Parke, Ross D., 150
Pipher, Mary, 151
Pollack, William S., 151
Sanger, Margaret, 152

Schwartz, Pepper, 153
Steinberg, Laurence D., 153
Tannen, Deborah, 154
Wallerstein, Judith S., 155
References, 156

6 **Facts and Data, 161**

7 **Directory of Organizations, Associations, and Agencies, 173**
Dating and Sexual Values, 173
Media Impact on Dating and Sexuality, 177
Internet Romance and Sex, 181
Dating and Club Drugs, 184
Date Rape, 188
Same-Sex Dating, 192
Premarital Sex, 195
Birth Control, 200
Teenage Pregnancy, 204
Sexually Transmitted Diseases, 208
Living Together, 212
Teenage Marriages, 215
Dating and Sexuality Education, 219

8 **Selected Print and Nonprint Resources, 223**
Part I: Books, 223
    Dating and Sexual Values, 223
    Media Impact on Dating and Sexuality, 226
    Internet Romance and Sex, 228
    Dating and Club Drugs, 230
    Date Rape, 232
    Same-Sex Dating, 234
    Premarital Sex, 237
    Birth Control, 239
    Teenage Pregnancy, 240
    Sexually Transmitted Diseases, 243
    Living Together, 245
    Teenage Marriages, 247
    Dating and Sexuality Education, 248
Part II: Journals and Online Publications, 250
Part III: Videos, 255

Glossary, 267
Index, 273
About the Author, 288

Preface

Few people can thrive on loneliness or isolation. Instead, most men and women begin dating by the time they reach adolescence, and in some cases, even sooner. The dynamics surrounding coupling in the United States have intrigued social scientists for years, and this important reference book is designed to share their findings. In the pages that follow, light is shed on how dating begins and endures, as well as how sexual attitudes and behaviors impact intimacy. Readers will receive an opportunity to better understand the dynamics of dating while simultaneously learning how to construct worthwhile and satisfying relationships with others.

Dating and sexuality in the United States have markedly changed since the past century, presenting modern teenagers with tremendous tests and challenges. Never has there been a greater need for teenagers, parents, educators, and social scientists to better understand dating and sexuality as it exists in modern life. As promiscuous sexual attitudes and behaviors are relentlessly transmitted to the young by the media, as cyberspace romance and dating have added new dimensions to Internet connections, as rates of sexually transmitted diseases among teens continue to soar, and as experiences such as "coed sleepovers" and "club drugs" have become part of the dating scene, society must discover ways to help young people find their way and make responsible choices.

This book speaks to such important needs in a candid, nonthreatening, straightforward way. Unfortunately, other books have presented topics such as sexually transmitted diseases and teen pregnancy in threatening or intimidating ways. That is not the case here. There is no attempt to be encyclopedic; rather, the "facts" of the book are interesting, informative, and readable. The result is a volume that supplies thought-provoking coverage of dating and sexuality: its basic trends, its concepts and problems, and its important issues and controversies.

The organizational framework of *Dating and Sexuality in America* consists of eight separate but interrelated chapters. The first chapter gives readers a historical overview of dating and sexuality in the United States, with a particular emphasis on changes that have occurred over the past century. Chapter 2 probes an assortment of important problems, controversies, and solutions related to dating and sexuality. The third chapter further discusses those issues and controversies from a worldwide perspective. Chapter 4 contains a brief, annotated chronological listing of major trends and events shaping dating and sexuality in the United States. And Chapter 5, biographical in design, complements the previous chapter by looking at the influential contributions of noteworthy social science researchers who shaped those trends. The sixth chapter provides important facts and data, and the seventh chapter includes a diverse and comprehensive directory of organizations, associations, and agencies. Chapter 8 offers readers recommended print resources such as journals and books, as well as nonprint resources such as films and videotapes. A glossary and index conclude the volume (with the exception of book titles, italic type denotes terms that are listed in the glossary).

The volume is designed for a broad range of readers in college, high school, and public library settings. It makes a valuable reference source for high school courses focusing on family life education, health education, or interpersonal relationships. At the college level, it has significant appeal to those students studying intimate relationships, human sexuality, adolescent development, gender issues, sexuality education, social psychology, and adjustment psychology.

Acknowledgments

Many people helped make this book a reality and deserve recognition. At Mitchell College, I extend appreciation to Dr. Mary Ellen Jukoski, Dr. Jane Friedrichs, and the Promotion Committee for granting me a sabbatical leave for research and writing purposes. Also at Mitchell College, I wish to thank Catherine Wright, Nancy Levine, David Brailey, Jennifer Mauro, Suzanne Risley, Steve Gruchawka, Laura Battista, Lindsay Bloom, and Katie Cichon for their assistance in locating and/or providing needed resources. I extend special appreciation to Lindsae Raineau for researching and writing the media influences in the dating section that appears in Chapter 2. I also thank the Alan Guttmacher Institute, the Annie E. Casey Foundation, the Population Reference Bureau, UNAIDS, and the United States Census Bureau for sharing their important research databases and assorted publications.

I have forged many new friendships at ABC-CLIO and wish to thank a truly outstanding team of publishing professionals. Acquisitions Editor Mim Vasan proved invaluable in shaping the direction of the project, particularly the book's identification of important dating issues and themes. The input and assistance of Editorial Assistant Jessica Bothwell was present from beginning to end, and her sunny disposition was always evident. Copyeditor Raven Moore Amerman worked tirelessly on the entire manuscript and, in addition to creating a smoother writing style, was responsible for many valuable text additions, improvements, and refinements. Finally, production editor Carla Roberts directed the transition from manuscript to book with consummate skill and was a joy to work with throughout the production process. Carla was a constant source of advice and enthusiasm and without her energy and ideas this project never would have materialized. It is to her honor that I dedicate *Dating and Sexuality in America.*

1

Background and History

This is a book about *dating*, the social process by which two people meet, interact, and pair off as a couple. The pages that follow will explore how dating has come to serve a number of important functions and purposes. For example, on the surface, dating provides companionship, as well as a vehicle for entertainment and recreation. Over the course of time, dating has become a social means for individuals to learn more about themselves and how they are perceived by others, who observe their strengths as well as weaknesses. Dating also teaches the importance of sharing and enables individuals to experience love and sexual activity within mutually acceptable limits. Finally, dating is the process through which one may ultimately select a marriage partner or other lifestyle.

Before launching into the book's focus, dating and sexuality of adolescents in the contemporary United States, some demographic information is useful. (For those readers seeking information on the intimate relationships of older adults, a number of important and worthwhile publications exist [e.g., L'Abate and DeGiacomo, 2003; Fletcher, 2002; Degenova and Rice, 2001; Ellis and Crawford, 2000].)

- Adolescents between the ages of 10 and 19 number approximately 39 million, and this figure is expected to rise to about 50 million by the year 2040.
- However, as a proportion of the total population, adolescents are projected to comprise only 13 percent of the total population by the year 2020, down from 14 percent in 2000.

- By 2040, the percentage of whites in the adolescent population will drop below 50 percent. Hispanics, on the other hand, are becoming the second most populous racial/ethnic group after non-Hispanic whites. Asian/Pacific Islanders, though small in number, have exhibited the fastest growth rate.
- About 20 percent of all adolescents live in poverty, and this figure is higher among black and Hispanic teens.
- There has been a dramatic decrease in the percentage of adolescents living in two-parent households. This decrease is fairly even across racial and ethnic groups. Children and adolescents ages 6–17 living in households with only their mother present are about five times as likely to be living in poverty than those living in two-parent households (U.S. Bureau of the Census, 2003).

People's present-day attitudes and behaviors related to dating did not spring up overnight. The socialization of both women and men in traditional gender roles and the restriction of sex to a procreative function within the institution of marriage are themes deeply embedded in time. Similarly, people's beliefs about such topics as sexual values, premarital sex, birth control, and alternative lifestyles also share a long and complex history.

Dating is common in most societies today, and variations of it have always existed, such as those related to traditions and customs. From the outset of this discussion, one must keep in mind that dating, at least in part, represents an extension and reflection of cultural beliefs and practices. *Culture* refers to everything individuals do or have as members of society. Culture serves to identify, organize, and unify people who share a common way of life.

More importantly, what is culturally important for one group of people may not even exist in another. Consider how perceived attractiveness varies from culture to culture, particularly how the body is altered in some way to make it conform to aesthetic or erotic ideals. For example, many Padaung women of Burma practice neck stretching because an elongated neck is considered graceful and attractive. Other cultures, such as those located in sub-Saharan Africa or Indonesia, maintain that physical beauty is enhanced when the ears, nose, and lips are pierced or perforated. In such societies, stretched lips and earlobes, filed teeth, and flattened skulls are also considered attractive.

Other dating and marriage practices further illustrate the

world of differences that exist. Kissing, although popular in the Western world, is not very widespread among the Japanese and Chinese. Among the Ainu of northern Japan and the Miao of mainland Asia, it is actually frowned upon. In some societies (e.g., parts of Asia, India, and Saudi Arabia), dating as Americans know it and the concept of choice does not exist; rather, the choice of a marriage partner is dictated or arranged by parents or some other authority. In China, the bride's dress is red—the color of love and joy—unlike the traditional white in the United States. And, although the Amish bride wears white at her wedding, it is for the first and only time in her life.

Such dating and mating variations, although admittedly quite different from our own in this country, do not suggest that those who practice them are inferior or strange. Different does not mean deficient, particularly when it comes to the concept of cultural relativism. *Cultural relativism* is the belief that there is no universal standard of good or bad when evaluating cultures. Any element of culture is deemed meaningful in relation to a particular location, time, and set of circumstances. One of the primary intentions of this book is to help foster a sensitive and tolerant understanding of the cultural variations that exist in regard to dating and sexuality. To help promote cultural relativism, chapter 3 (Worldwide Perspective) offers important international perspectives on these topics.

Just as some worldwide customs might seem strange to people outside those particular cultures, some of the dating and sexual behaviors practiced in this country or some of the problems related to dating may seem unusual or downright strange to those seeking to understand American culture: cyberspace romances, coed sleepovers, acquaintance rape, and club drugs, to name but a few. Some of American teens' problems seem to defy legitimate explanations, particularly when one places them against the backdrop of this country's international status. For instance, why do American teenagers, who live in one of the most powerful and educationally sophisticated nations on Earth, have the dubious distinction of being among the world's leaders in rates of teenage pregnancy, births, abortion, and sexually transmitted diseases? (Problems and issues such as these will receive full attention in chapter 2.)

And, if eyebrows were raised at the discussion above of some of the body modifications and alterations practiced in other cultures, keep in mind that American teenagers have their own unique definitions and displays of physical attractiveness and distinctiveness. For some teenagers, it is exhibited in nontraditional fashions, such as oversized clothing, NFL team jerseys, or Iraqi Freedom camouflage. For others, hair is a sign of distinctiveness, from a rainbow of colorings, to corn braiding and dreadlocks, to shaven heads. For still others, attractiveness is a more permanent alteration, such as a body tattoo, branding, or piercing. Body jewelry and ornaments usually prompt a second glance: tongue studs and barbells, nipple rings, navel rings, nose and eyebrow jewelry, to name some of the more common. Other teenagers take more drastic measures like altering their looks through fad diets to look unrealistically thin or through implants and injections to acquire the perfect body contour. Certainly, American teenagers are culturally different from their cohorts around the globe and are a reflection of their place and time in history.

How can one explain such behaviors? How did dating evolve to its present-day form in the United States? How do today's practices and trends compare to those of the past? This chapter will seek to answer such questions by taking a walk back through time. Social scientists have a fairly good picture of how dating and sexual behavior have evolved in the United States. Time and space preclude offering an analysis of the entire United States' history, but this book can touch on some of the major developments occurring at key points: the early 1900s, the Roaring Twenties, World War II, the sexual revolution, and the twenty-first century. Examining these historical eras will enable readers to discover some interesting variations in teenage dating and sexual behaviors: courtship customs and traditions, gender roles, sexual promiscuity, contraception, and marriage trends, among them. While some dating behaviors and sexual attitudes have remained fairly constant over time, others have changed considerably.

The Early 1900s

The United States at the turn of the twentieth century was a nation experiencing great change. The government brought about important, progressive changes at this time, such as enacting women's suffrage, improving working conditions, restricting child labor, and creating educational reform. Industrialism was very much a part of the national landscape, particularly in the eastern regions, where urban populations swelled. Europeans were immigrating to this country in unprecedented numbers: between 1900 and 1910, almost 10 million immigrants entered the United States. Considerable migration also took place within the nation. Many farmers were leaving the relentless demands of the fields for what they believed to be an easier and more prosperous life in the city. More modern farm machinery contributed to the rural exodus: vast numbers of laborers were no longer needed to produce the basic food supply. As workers abandoned the plow in favor of the factory, the relative importance of city and farm in the United States changed forever (Beaudoin, 2003; Fitzgerald, 2003).

Teenagers growing up at the turn of the century would be impacted by the many social changes ushered in by industrialization. For example, the combination of foreign and domestic immigrants to the cities brought new ideologies and traditions. Cultures from old and established European nations, in particular, made Americans more aware of differences in religion, politics, and economics. As a result of this cultural infusion, attitudes about such topics as dating and courtship, the idealization of women, the concept of romantic love, and gender issues were compared and contrasted.

Industrialization created shifts in family functioning, such as economic well being, which in turn entrenched traditional gender role behaviors. Instead of functioning together as a productive agrarian unit, families now seldom worked together physically. In the growing number of nonfarm families, the husband/father went off to work in an industrial setting while the wife/mother stayed at home with the children. Thus, an important variation in gender role behaviors occurred. Women, once partners in labor in farming families, were now exclusively assigned to the home and the hearth. Although small numbers of women entered the labor force, employment outside of the home and away from the family became the province of the man.

The turn of the century also marked a time when most American and European cultures liberated themselves from rigid Victorian attitudes about sex. *Victorianism* occurred during the middle to late 1800s and reflected a time when sex was regarded as a taboo. It was a time of heightened morality and a repressive attitude toward sexuality. The topic of sex was shrouded in silence or whispers, especially in public, and many people tried to pretend that sexual desire did not exist. In so doing, anxiety, guilt, shame, and confusion compounded each other as Victorians struggled to achieve the high morality they envisioned.

While the Victorian veil of sexual repression began to erode, traditional gender roles remained, and they prescribed the behaviors and expectations of men and women. Men were expected to be assertive, dominant, and in control. They were expected to postpone marriage until they had established themselves in the vocational world. Women, on the other hand, were taught to be subservient, dependent, and submissive. They were expected to be passive and nonaggressive, and to subordinate their needs to those exhibited by men (Inglehart and Norris, 2003; Langland, 2002).

Traditional gender role expectations would also dictate the course of dating and sexual behaviors in the future. Indeed, the traditional expectations held for men and women would create what is referred to as a *cultural role script*, a preconception of how one should behave in a social setting. A cultural role script creates an image that instructs people about appropriate goals, desirable qualities, and typical behaviors. Related to dating, the traditional role script dictates that the man initiate courtship behaviors, including asking the woman out, covering the financial expenses of the date, and supplying transportation to and from the dating activity.

The traditional cultural role script also defines what sexual behaviors are right or wrong, as well as the level of involvement each partner should have. Men are seen as the initiators of sexual intimacy as well as of whatever sexual escalation is to take place. Even though Victorian attitudes about sex were changing during this era, the United States at the turn of the century was still very much a sexually conservative nation. Unmarried couples were expected to remain abstinent and to refrain from sexual activity until marriage vows were exchanged. Of course, whether or not couples did or didn't follow this convention would intrigue human sexuality researchers for decades.

Cultural role scripts were handed down from generation to generation and were taught in many different ways. Books describing the "proper" behavior for men and women to follow were available, including Emily Post's *Etiquette in Society, in Business, in Politics and at Home* (1922). Post's book was extremely popular, and her advice reflects society's preferred images of masculinity and femininity at that time. Consider, for example, her advice on social etiquette for men: "A gentleman always rises when a lady comes into a room. In public places men do not jump up for every strange woman who happens to approach. But if any woman addresses a remark to him, a gentleman at once rises to his feet as he answers her" (p. 38).

Post's fashion advice to women of the day: " . . . walking on the street—if you care to be taken for a well-bred person—never wear anything that is exaggerated. If skirts are short, don't wear them two inches shorter than any one else's . . . Don't wear too much jewelry; it is in bad taste in the first place, and in the second, is a temptation to a thief. And don't under any circumstances, distort your figure into a grotesque shape" (p. 46).

The cultural role script of the times called for structured and rather formal dating arrangements, and longer courtship periods were more common than shorter ones. The man took the initiative to ask the woman out (as mentioned previously), and this had to be done well in advance of the date. The man often "called upon" the woman in person to request her company, a social exchange that served the added purpose of providing parents with an opportunity to meet the suitor. Dating activities often included dining out, dancing, attending a church social, or some other neighborhood recreational activity. It was not uncommon for a parent or other designated adult to chaperone a date. Couples often opted to spend the evening in the woman's residence, which spared expenses but obviously limited privacy if she lived with her parents. The assembly-line production of the Model T automobile in 1908 introduced mobility and privacy into the dating lives of couples. Now, couples could be together beyond the watchful eyes of parents.

The United States' involvement in World War I was relatively short (1917–1918), particularly when compared to the many long years of combat that would accompany other wars (e.g., World War II, Korean War, Cambodian War). However, World War I still impacted society in various ways, including changes in dating and cultural role scripts. Because no one knew at the time how long World War I would last, courtship periods tended to be brief, and dating became less structured and formal. Although research on sexual behavior during this time is scant, it is likely that more sexual freedom characterized relationships. As dating partners, fiancés, and spouses were shipped off to Europe, the durability of relationships and the fidelity of partners was put to the test. Love letters exchanged between soldiers and their romantic partners took on new meaning and importance. On the home front, World War I brought a shift in gender roles. Because women's labor was critically needed outside the home, the societal separation of work and family life became blurred. And thousands of women joined the armed forces, creating further variations of the cultural role script.

A few trends in marriage and family life in the early 1900s might be noted here. Regarding the median age at first marriage for the entire population, in 1900 it was 23.9 (21.9 for women and 25.9 for men), and in 1910 it dipped to 23.3 (21.6 for women and 25.1 for men). Regarding the nation's *fertility rate* (the number of children that a woman can be expected to have over the course of her reproductive life), between 1900 and 1910 it stood at about 3.5 (U.S. Bureau of the Census, 2003; National Center for Health Statistics, 2001). For a statistical portrait of median ages at first marriage from 1900 to 2000 and fertility rates from 1910 to 2000, refer to chapter 6, table 6.2 and figure 6.1.

The "Roaring Twenties"

Our nation's future never seemed brighter than when the United States entered the "Roaring Twenties," a colorful and exciting decade in American history. American cities continued to mushroom, and the prospect of economic opportunity drew millions of immigrants from abroad. The country's transformation into an industrial giant brought a wave of unprecedented prosperity, including the emergence of a consumer culture. Americans were in search of an easier and better life, and modern household conveniences showed that progress was being made, including inventions like the refrigerator, washing machine, electric toaster, and air conditioning. The rising popularity of the automobile, which growing numbers of people could now afford, seemed to capture the self-indulgence of the times as well as an America on the go. The success of Henry Ford's Model T was a case in point: between 1908 and 1927, more than 18 million of these automobiles had rolled off the assembly lines (Gourley, 1997).

Teenagers growing up in the 1920s witnessed further liberation from Victorian sexual restraints, and they experienced a revolution in morals and manners. Women, in particular, achieved new levels of autonomy and freedom. In 1920, the Nineteenth Amendment to the Constitution, granting women the right to vote, was signed into law. Those women working outside the home established some degree of financial independence and were exposed to a wider pool of potential dating partners. Furthermore, the sexual needs and sexual rights of women were being increasingly recognized. The image of the shy, dependent, and passive woman was being eroded.

Independent and daring young "flappers" were among those rewriting the traditional cultural role scripts for women. Flappers were young women who wore short skirts and revealing outfits, smoked and drank, and danced into the night in social clubs called "speakeasies." The drinking of alcoholic beverages was outlawed at the time by Prohibition laws, which sought to prevent the manufacture, transportation, and sale of alcoholic beverages. However, singles and couples alike found their way to these local "speakeasies" and consumed illegal alcohol. Such behavior represents an interesting historical variation of the illegal drug consumption of today's teenagers. Although the drug of choice has changed in modern times, one can only wonder if the underlying behavior and motives have not remained the same.

Parental control over courtship lessened considerably during this time, and arranged marriages became a thing of the past for the majority of couples. The automobile continued to supply couples with a means to escape the prying eyes of parents and other family members. Women experienced much more freedom in selecting a mate, and for most partners of both sexes, love and affection became pivotal features of the relationship. The concept of romantic love was reborn and became increasingly popular. Also, the public was exposed to new thoughts and interpretations of human sexuality, including the psychoanalytic theory of Sigmund Freud (see chapter 5).

During the 1920s, birth control activists spoke out, established clinics, and distributed information about contraception methods. Abstinence, withdrawal, the condom, and abortion were the most widely used methods of birth control, but other contraceptive measures such as the intrauterine device (IUD) were under development. One of the more outspoken activists at the time was Margaret Sanger, an instrumental figure in the American birth control movement. A nurse, Sanger wrote and distributed booklets on birth control and opened clinics to advise people on methods and techniques. Because it was illegal to distribute birth control information, Sanger, who was responsible for founding the Planned Parenthood Federation of America, was arrested many times. (A biographical sketch of Sanger's life can be found in chapter 5.)

The economic prosperity that seemed so promising at the beginning of the 1920s proved to be short-lived, however. Indeed, the fact that such prosperity was unevenly distributed and that it excluded farmers and unskilled workers was one of the major factors contributing to the collapse of the American economy. The stock market crash of October 1929 precipitated the Great Depression, which lasted for the next ten years and brought unprecedented unemployment and poverty to the nation. Between 1932 and 1933, 16 million workers became unemployed—approximately one-quarter of the available labor force—and industrial production dropped off by 50 percent (James, 2002; McElvaine, 1993).

Dating and courtship, as well as marriage and family life, during the Great Depression mirrored the grim economics of the time. Vast numbers of Americans found themselves homeless and even penniless. Courtships were often interrupted as families frequently moved about the country to find any kind of work they could. When dating took place, the cultural role script was dictated by frugality and financial vigilance. Regarding couples' dating activities, most simply could not afford gasoline for their automobiles (if they owned one), public transportation costs (if a system was available), or expenditures for entertainment and recreational activities. Family outings, town-sponsored events such as dances, or simply enjoying the company of each other were common activities. Much like society as a whole, the couple relationship was characterized by the time-honored virtues of thrift and hard work.

As far as the median age at first marriage was concerned, in 1920 it was 22.9 (21.2 for women and 24.6 for men), and in 1930 it was 22.8 (21.3 for women and 24.3 for men). The Great Depression also impacted family planning. At one time, large families had been encouraged because children were perceived as making worthwhile and productive contributions to the family unit. Now, children became economic liabilities, as parents had more mouths to feed in their daily struggles to carve out an existence. The fertility rate stood at 3.3 during the early 1920s but dropped to 2.2 during the Great Depression. The percentage of childless marriages also increased (Population Reference Bureau, 2002a; National Center for Health Statistics, 2001).

World War II

World War II, which began for the United States in 1941 and lasted until 1945, involved every major power in the world. It killed more people and damaged more property than any other war in history had up to that point. It is estimated that 70 million people served in the armed forces during the war. As far as military casualties were concerned, more than 17 million combatants died, 400,000 of these being Americans. Seventy nations participated in World War II, and combat took place in Europe, Asia, and Africa and in the seas surrounding Australia (Hoopes, 2002).

World War II exerted a tremendous impact on American life. As men were sent off to war, women took their places in the workplace, especially in war plants. Although increasing numbers of women had entered the labor force during the past few decades, World War II sparked the first great exodus of women from the home to the workplace. By 1943, more than 2 million women were employed in American war industries. Overall, about 6.3 million women entered the labor force during World War II (Lewis, 2002; Klam, 2002).

"Rosie the Riveter" captured the image of the wartime female employee: skilled, strong, patriotic, and dependable. Within the labor force, women acquired new vocational skills, established financial freedom, and were no longer expected to fulfill traditional gender role behaviors. Though most women had to relinquish their jobs to the men returning home when World War II ended, they had tasted independence and had done their part to help win the war.

World War II affected dating and courtship in many ways. Much like World War I, the war separated lovers for extended periods of time, and it therefore tested the limits of relationships' durability and partners' fidelity. On the home front, courtships were often brief, and more permissive sexual attitudes and behaviors became evident. Many women seemed more independent and self-sufficient, behaviors likely due to their greater labor-force participation. Men serving in the armed forces came in contact with women from different parts of the country and different parts of the world. Many men serving in the armed forces married women from other nations, some choosing to return home with their new family members while others opted to settle overseas. At home, female employees working in wartime industrial settings met increasing numbers of eligible dating partners, many from different parts of the United States. In short, people met dating partners from increasingly different walks of life. Such changing scenarios captured how a different dimension of dating and courtship in the United States had been set in motion. As with the infusion of immigrants at the turn of the century, many Americans became exposed to wide multicultural differences.

When the war ended, a victorious United States was in a celebratory mood. Between 1945 and 1953, more than 10 million men and women were released from the armed services. America's heroes had returned, and the nation's freedom had been protected. All embraced peace, and stability was restored to civilian life. Men and women now wanted to live the American dream—find a job, buy a car, marry, raise a family, and buy a house. Although some feared that the nation might return to the stark economic times characterizing the 1930s, such pessimism proved unfounded. Indeed, the postwar United States experienced a dramatic economic boom and a period of sustained prosperity. While much of the world lay in devastated ruin and financial upheaval, the United States enjoyed unparalleled economic security (Zinn, 2002).

The postwar dating scene reflected the affluence of the times. No longer were adolescents expected to financially support their families, nor were they shipped off to war; indeed, teenagers enjoyed more freedom and leisure time than ever before. A new chapter of dating and courtship in the United States was written, one that seemed to mirror the spirit of the nation. Just as earlier generations of teenagers had left their mark, so too did the adolescents of the 1950s: fast cars, drive-in movie theaters, going steady, and sock hops. Rock and roll, a distinctive music style triggering a flurry of new dance steps, was introduced to an entire nation, and inventions such as transistor radios, 45-rpm records, and color television broadcasts found their way into homes that would never quite be the same. The United States was at peace and at play.

Although sexual attitudes and behaviors were still on the conservative and traditional side, the United States was beginning to exhibit more curiosity about the topic of sex and a desire to learn more about its many sides. While the value of Sigmund Freud's psychoanalytical theory was being weighed and the family planning measures advocated by Margaret Sanger were being debated, other inroads to human sexuality were being developed. Among the more notable contributions at this time was the research of Alfred Kinsey, who undertook the nation's first truly comprehensive survey of sexual behavior. No one before Kinsey had dared to ask so many people so many direct and detailed questions about their intimate sexual behaviors, and the general public eagerly awaited the results (Kinsey's biographical sketch and a discussion of his research can be found in chapter 5).

The wedding bells rang for Americans when the war was over. In 1946, about 2.2 million couples exchanged wedding vows, which was quite a jump from the 1.6 million in 1945. This total would represent the nation's highest number of marriages until 1979, when 2.3 million couples would go to the altar. In 1945, about 9 percent of the unions involved teenagers, and the average age at marriage was 22.2 (21.2 for women and 23.2 for men) (U.S. Bureau of the Census, 2003; National Center for Health Statistics, 2001; Population Reference Bureau, 2000).

It should be pointed out, too, that divorce rates skyrocketed in the postwar United States. In 1946, 610,000 divorces were granted, a significant increase from the 485,000 marriages dissolved in 1945. This would remain the high-water mark for divorces until 1969, at which time 639,000 divorces would be granted (U.S. Bureau of the Census, 2003).

This generation also proved to be a very fertile one, particularly between the years 1946 (the fertility rate was 3.1) and 1964 (3.6). During this time span, the nation would experience an explosion of births, prompting demographers to label this time period the *baby boom.* "Baby boomers," as they came to be known, were born between 1946 and 1964 and today number approximately 76 million (about 30 percent of the population). Reasons for the baby boom are, of course, speculative. However, one would think that seeking to fulfill the previously mentioned American dream, along with youthful optimism and an increased emphasis placed on family, were important motivating factors (Population Reference Bureau, 2002a).

The baby boom became evident in 1946, when births went from 2.8 million in 1945 to 3.4 million. The peak boom year was 1957, when 4.3 million infants were born (see chapter 6, table 6.3). The ratio of boys to girls remained relatively constant during the boom: approximately 1.05 male births for every one female birth. As far as ethnicity is concerned, 61 million of the boomers were white, 9 million African American, and 6 million Hispanic American, Asian American, or Native American (U.S. Bureau of the Census, 2003; Population Reference Bureau, 2002a; National Center for Health Statistics, 2001).

The Sexual Revolution

The winds of change were strong in the late 1960s as the conservatism of the 1950s gave way to revolutionary styles of thinking. The 1960s represented a time when approximately 70 million children from the 1950s baby boom generation became adolescents and young adults. This population cohort became a liberal and outspoken breed, one that challenged the conventional culture of the times. The new generation—unique in dress, language, and its own brand of music—scorned materialism and sought social change on many fronts, including values, lifestyles, and laws. The generation's methods of protest, from sit-ins to protest marches, took place against the backdrop of significant historical events: the assassination of John F. Kennedy, civil rights protests, the Vietnam War, and Watergate.

Because many of the changes that occurred at this time involved sexuality, social scientists labeled the 1960s the sexual revolution. *Sexual revolution* refers to changes in thinking about human sexuality that focused on gender roles as well as specifically on sexual behavior. The sexual revolution introduced changes that helped to mold contemporary sexual attitudes and behaviors: a shift in relations between men and women, the continuing and accentuating commercialization of sex, changes in the ways sexual behavior is regulated, the emergence of new social antagonisms, and the appearance of new political movements (Kamen, 2002; Allyn, 2001).

The controversy surrounding the sexual revolution has produced many interpretations of the era and the phenomena that have characterized it. One interpretation is that the sexual revolution brought about more relaxed and tolerant attitudes and a more flexible morality. Another is that it brought about greater equality, both general and sexual, between men and women. Yet another interpretation takes a dim view of the so-called liberation of women during the sexual revolution and regards it instead as largely a myth. Although many women today hold managerial and leadership positions, this interpretation holds that most women remain trapped in low-paying jobs, have few career opportunities, and, in addition, shoulder most of the burden of child care.

There is no mistaking the fact that teenagers growing up during the sexual revolution witnessed vivid eruptions of sexual display. For example, many movie and rock stars began to present themselves in a highly erotic fashion through their appearance, dress, and movements on stage and in the lyrics of their songs. In major cities, commercialized sex—for example, prostitution and the sale of pornographic materials—grew rapidly. Attitudes toward contraception, divorce, abortion, premarital and extramarital sex, cohabitation, and homosexuality relaxed somewhat. The

1960s also saw a huge change in the openness with which sexual matters were discussed (Reiss and Ellis, 2002).

The media played a significant role in influencing sexual values. For example, a growing movement away from traditional morality became apparent. Bans on books were removed and Hollywood movies contained more sexually suggestive themes. A number of Supreme Court decisions of the 1960s and 1970s were influential in promoting more liberal sexual attitudes. For example, the Court ruled that graphic discussion and depiction of sexual acts was protected by the constitutional right of free speech. Although standards of enforcement varied from state to state, sexually explicit books, magazines, and films became widely available.

Even some of the human sexuality research of the day had a certain daring and boldness to it. In the mid-1960s, William Masters and Virginia Johnson created public and professional stirrings by scientifically studying in the laboratory such sexual activities as masturbation and sexual intercourse (see chapter 5). Their book, *Human Sexual Response* (1966), became a runaway best-seller, its success reflecting the growing curiosity and interest of the times.

Complete frontal nudity of both men and women was no longer restricted to hard-core pornography but now began to appear in such over-the-counter magazines as *Playboy* and *Cosmopolitan*. Sex manuals also found their way onto bookstore shelves, offering readers an assortment of sexual pleasuring techniques. In the world of advertising, sex was used in more direct ways to promote a diversity of products, from blue jeans to sports cars.

The sexual revolution succeeded in ushering in a new era of adolescent dating and sexual behavior. Compared to earlier decades, dating became a less structured activity and took on a more casual and spontaneous quality. For many, traditional gender role attitudes and behaviors began to erode and were replaced with more sharing and equity between dating partners.

As far as sexual values were concerned, growing numbers of adolescents, particularly college students, moved away from the *abstinence orientation* (it is morally wrong for unmarried persons to engage in sexual relations) in favor of the *permissiveness with affection orientation* (premarital sexual relations are morally acceptable, provided there is emotional attachment between partners). Some couples adopted the *permissiveness without affection* or *hedo-*

nistic orientation. Unlike the permissiveness with affection orientation, the hedonistic orientation views intercourse by itself (without emotional attachment) as acceptable (see chapter 2 for a discussion of all sexual standards). Because of these shifts in sexual standards, rates of premarital intercourse increased from those of earlier years.

In relation to the increase of sexual activity, a few statistics are warranted. When Alfred Kinsey conducted his postwar surveys on human sexuality (Kinsey, Pomeroy, and Martin, 1948; Kinsey et al., 1953), he discovered that 20 percent of the women queried and 40 percent of the men had experienced sexual intercourse by the time they were age 20. An investigation conducted by Robertson Sorensen (1973) concerned the sexual behavior of males and females between the ages of 13 and 19. Among his findings, it was discovered that 59 percent of the males studied and 45 percent of the females had engaged in sexual intercourse at least once. Furthermore, a substantial percentage of the respondents had experienced intercourse at earlier ages than reported by Kinsey. Yet, although percentages had increased, Sorensen found that in most cases, those engaging in premarital sex were doing so with only one partner to whom they felt emotionally close, a reflection of the emerging permissiveness with affection value orientation.

Improved birth control methods during the sexual revolution also contributed to increases in adolescent sexual activity. For example, in 1960, the FDA approved the birth control pill (oral contraceptive), and in 1963, the intrauterine device (IUD) became widely available. Because of the birth control pill especially, the fear of pregnancy was lessened. However, as will be further discussed in chapter 2, a birth control device such as the Pill offers no protection against sexually transmitted diseases (STDs), which began increasing among teens during the sexual revolution. Also, despite the fact that many birth control options were now available, many teenagers still engaged in unprotected sexual activity, both then and now.

Teenage pregnancy and abortion were other results of adolescents' increased sexual activity. During the sexual revolution, adolescent pregnancy rates rose. For example, in 1970, more than 660,000 births were from mothers under 20 years of age, one of the highest teen birth totals ever. The rates remained fairly steady through the 1980s and mid-1990s (around 520,000 per year), then they began to decline. Abortion was made legal at the height of the sexual revolution in 1973 in the landmark court case of *Roe v. Wade*. Abortion rates rose during the sexual revolution (about 380,000), held fairly constant during the 1980s (about 350,000), and then began a steady decline (Population Reference Bureau, 2000; 2002a). Several reasons can be cited for the decline in adolescent pregnancy, birth, and abortion rates. Declines in teenagers' level of sexual activity and continued increases in their use and effective use of contraceptives are major reasons. Chapter 2 explores each of these areas.

As far as rates of teenage marriage during the sexual revolution were concerned, in 1960, about 9.1 percent of all marriages involved adolescents, but this figure fell to about 7.2 percent in 1970, and then dipped again to 5.1 percent by 1980. Regarding the median age at first marriage for the entire population, in 1960 it was 21.5 (20.3 for women and 22.8 for men), in 1970 it rose to 22.0 (20.8 for women and 23.2 for men), and it increased to 23.3 in 1980 (22.0 for women and 24.7 for men). Regarding the nation's fertility rate during the sexual revolution, in 1960 it stood at 3.6, it dropped to 2.5 in 1970, and it fell again in 1980 to around 2.0 (U.S. Bureau of the Census, 2003).

The Twenty-First Century

The nature of contemporary adolescent dating and sexual behavior is the subject of this book, including the problems and controversies to be addressed in chapter 2. This section, then, will bring the historical chronology into the present by touching on some key trends and changes in dating and sexual behavior in more recent years. This will bring closure to this history chapter while simultaneously setting the stage for what follows.

In contrast to the baby boom generation of 1946–1964, teenagers born after 1964 and before 1980 are sometimes referred to as baby busters, or *Generation X*. The "baby busters" designation evolved as the nation's fertility rate sank between 1965 (3.5) and 1980 (1.9). (It should be noted that the generational names and time spans vary depending on the research consulted. Regarding the former, teens of the new millennium are called by some the "N-Generation" for *nanotechnology*.) Today, the fertility rate stands at just about 2.0. Members of Generation X see themselves as a unique cohort, one sharing historical, economic, and cultural experiences different from those of baby boomers and other generations. To illustrate, teenage Xers are very comfortable with using information and technology and tend to be creative, self-reliant workers. Readers seeking more information on Generation X are referred to Zemke, Raines, and Filipczak (2000); Raines (1997); and Thau (1997).

However one refers to today's generation of teenagers, researchers know that dating begins early, between 13 and 14 years of age for many. Similar to a trend starting in the sexual revolution, dating for the most part is not structured and formal; rather, it is more relaxed and spontaneous. Dating relationships often evolve out of relationships in adolescent peer groups, such as those originating from the school, neighborhood, or special interests (e.g., sports, religion, clubs). It is not uncommon for a couple to go out on a date within a larger group activity, such as a group of teens going to a shopping mall, movie, athletic event, or other type of school function.

One group activity connected to the dating scene that has increased in recent years is coed sleepovers. A *coed sleepover* is an overnight, mixed-gender gathering of teenagers in the home of one of the participants. The adolescents usually watch television, listen to music or rent videos, share party foods such as pizza, and then sleep on whatever bedding is available. When closely monitored and structured, such sleepovers are generally viewed by parents as permissible and a normal part of the adolescent socialization experience. However, some parents do not permit their teens to attend such activities; they feel that supervision is often too lax, which makes sexual exploration too tempting, particularly if alcohol and drugs are present.

Today's teenagers are greatly impacted by the media, including dating scenarios portrayed in television, films, and music. From television soap operas to sitcoms, from Hollywood "chick flicks" to MTV videos, media characters often serve as role models for adolescents to imitate, sometimes without even realizing it. Furthermore, as will be discussed in chapter 2, the media may have the effect, at least in part, for increasing sexual promiscuity in today's society and, by extension, among adolescents. Television in particular is easily accessible to teenagers, and in the minds of many researchers (e.g., Holtzman, 2000; Johnston and Fishman, 2000), it has changed the rules of what is seen as normal and acceptable. Critics such as Gunter (2002) and Dines and Humez (2002) maintain that the media has too much sexually suggestive content, which provides teens with a steady diet of titillation and examples of provocative behavior. (Subsequent sections of this book will explore the potentially negative effects that such sexual messages and images can have on teenagers especially and discuss ways to convey more realistic and appropriate images to modern Americans concerning dating relationships and sexuality.)

Compared to previous generations, teenagers of the twenty-first century have different ways to establish contact with their friends and dating partners, such as cell phones, pagers, and palm pilots. They also have a new way to meet partners unheard of by their predecessors: the Internet. The *Internet* is a large computer network linking smaller computer networks worldwide. Today, it is estimated that more than 167 million households are online, and adolescents are heavy users of the Internet (U.S. Bureau of the Census, 2003). Teenagers are often drawn to chat rooms by the lure of meeting different people and creating a cyberspace relationship (the term "cyberspace" refers to the realm of electronic communication). A *cyberspace romance* may result, that is, the formation of a romantic online relationship. Such relationships are not uncommon among teens, and neither are visitations to pornographic websites. Researchers (e.g., Fein and Schneider, 2002; Akdeniz, 2000) point out that it is important for parents to monitor adolescent computer romances as well as to restrict their children's access to pornography on the Internet, and to consider the degree to which computer monitoring and supervision should take place at home. The next chapter will revisit this topic.

As will also be discussed in the next chapter, most of today's adolescents are sexually active, and sexual activity begins at earlier ages than in the past. Such widespread rates of sexual activity create a number of health risks for today's adolescents, namely sexually transmitted diseases, pregnancy, and abortion. As far as STDs are concerned, today's teenagers are especially susceptible to contracting chlamydia and gonorrhea, and teenage cases of HIV/AIDS have been on the rise. In 2001, adolescent and adult women represented 26 percent of new AIDS cases, compared to only 11 percent in 1990 and 6 percent in 1982 (Population Reference Bureau, 2002b).

As far as unwed pregnancy is concerned, more than one million adolescent females become pregnant annually, and about half of this total give birth to their babies. Adolescent females are nearly three times as likely as adolescent males to become custodial parents. (Adolescent mothers and their babies—dubbed by some as "children having children"—face many health risks and other problems, which will be explored later in this book.) Also, in 2000, 1.3 million abortions took place, 19 percent of this total being abortions performed on adolescents (Alan Guttmacher Institute, 2002; Centers for Disease Control, 2000; 2001; Planned Parenthood Federation of America, 2001).

Finally, for those adolescents choosing to cohabit or marry, a few trends are noteworthy. Among older teenagers and young adults, cohabitation is a popular lifestyle option. (While definitions of *cohabitation* vary, it is generally recognized as the status reserved for couples who are unmarried, living in the same household, and who share certain obligations equivalent to a spousal-type relationship.) Approximately 5 million people chose to cohabit in 2000, a significant increase from the approximate one-half million choosing to do so in 1970. As far as adolescent marriages are concerned, about 4.5 of all marriages in 2000 involved teens, up slightly from the approximate 4 percent of teens who exchanged vows in 1990. Overall, the median age at first marriage in 2000 was 25.9 (25.1 for women and 26.8 for men) (U.S. Bureau of the Census, 2003; National Center for Health Statistics, 2001). The topics of cohabitation and teenage marriages will be revisited in chapter 2.

Summary

Dating and sexual behaviors are influenced by social conditions, cultural norms, and institutional structures. This chapter has traced the manner in which dating and sexual behavior have been impacted by unique periods in American history: the early 1900s, the Roaring Twenties, World War II, the sexual revolution, and the twenty-first century. Of course, any interpretation of history is selective and prone to oversimplification. Nevertheless, tracing the early beginnings of dating in the United States should show how today's dating and sexual expressions reflect a convergence of past influences. Indeed, as customs and conventions have changed or shifted in the United States, so too did the complexion of dating.

By exploring the past, readers' curiosity has hopefully been piqued about dating and sexuality in the new millennium and what the future may have in store for teenagers. Without question, dating and sexual behavior in the United States has changed over the course of the past century. Americans have witnessed greater levels of sexual freedom and more positive lifestyle options. But one must not lose sight of the fact that such changes have also been accompanied by new challenges and problems. For instance, sexual freedom, although seen as desirable among young people, often pushes them into relationships that they are unprepared to handle. Most are not ready for the emotional involvement or commitment that such relationships require, and not enough teens are provided with guidance to teach them relationship and family-life skills or to introduce them to the concepts of sexual responsibility and risk reduction. Adults need to provide ongoing educational opportunities on topics such as these so that adolescents can better understand themselves and those they date. In so doing, adolescents can live and grow to their fullest potential, and the relationships they forge will prosper.

References

Akdeniz, Yaman. 2000. *Sex on the Net: The Dilemma of Policing Cyberspace.* New York: South Street.

Alan Guttmacher Institute. 2002. *Sexual and Reproductive Health of Men and Women.* New York: Author.

Allyn, David. 2001. *Make Love, Not War: The Sexual Revolution: An Unfettered History.* Florence, KY: Routledge.

Beaudoin, Stephen. 2003. *Industrial Revolution.* Boston: Houghton Mifflin.

Centers for Disease Control. 2000. Division of Sexually Transmitted Diseases. *Sexually Transmitted Disease Surveillance.* Atlanta, GA: Author.

———. 2001. Division of Sexually Transmitted Diseases. *HIV/AIDS Surveillance Report.* Atlanta, GA: Author.

Degenova, Mary Kay, and E. Phillip Rice. 2001. *Intimate Relationships, Marriages, and Families.* New York: McGraw-Hill.

Dines, Gail, and Jean M. Humez, eds. 2002. *Gender, Race and Class in Media.* Thousand Oaks, CA: Sage.

Ellis, Albert, and Ted Crawford. 2000. *Making Intimate Connections: Seven Guidelines for Great Relationships and Better Communication.* San Francisco: Insight.

Fein, Ellen, and Sherrie Schneider. 2002. *The Rules for Online Dating.* New York: Simon and Schuster.

Fitzgerald, Deborah. 2003. *Every Farm a Factory: The Industrial Ideal in American Agriculture.* New Haven, CT: Yale University Press.

Fletcher, Garth. 2002. *The New Science of Intimate Relationships.* Williston, VT: Blackwell.

Gourley, Catherine. 1997. *Wheels of Time: A Biography of Henry Ford.* Brookfield, CT: Millbrook.

Gunter, Barrie. 2002. *Media Sex: What Are the Issues?* Mahwah, NJ: Lawrence Erlbaum.

Holtzman, Linda. 2000. *What Film, Television, and Popular Music Teach Us about Race, Class, Gender and Sexual Orientation.* Armonk, NY: M. E. Sharpe.

Hoopes, Roy. 2002. *Americans Remember the Home Front: An Oral Narrative of the World War II Years in America.* East Rutherford, NJ: Berkley.

Inglehart, Ronald, and Pippa Norris. 2003. *Gender Equality and Cultural Change around the World.* Portchester, NY: Cambridge University Press.

James, Harold. 2002. *The End to Globalization: Lessons from the Great Depression.* Cambridge, MA: Harvard University Press.

Johnston, Carla B., and Donald Fishman. 2000. *Screened Out: How the Media Control Us and What We Can Do about It.* Armonk, NY: M. E. Sharpe.

Kamen, Paula. 2002. *Her Way: Young Women Remake the Sexual Revolution.* NY: Broadway.

Kinsey, Alfred. C., Wardell B. Pomeroy, and Clyde E. Martin. 1948. *Sexual Behavior in the Human Male.* Philadelphia: W. B. Saunders.

Kinsey, Alfred. C., Wardell B. Pomeroy, Clyde E. Martin, and Paul H. Gebhard. 1953. *Sexual Behavior in the Human Female.* Philadelphia: W. B. Saunders.

Klam, Julie. 2002. *War at Home.* New York: Smart Apple Media.

L'Abate, Luciano, and Piero DeGiacomo. 2003. *Intimate Relationships and How to Improve Them.* Westport, CT: Greenwood.

Langland, Elizabeth. 2002. *Telling Tales: Essays on Gender and Narrative Form in Victorian Literature and Culture.* Columbus, OH: Ohio State University Press.

Lewis, Brenda R. 2002. *Women at War: The Women in World War II, at Home, at Work, on the Front Line.* East Rutherford, NJ: Putnam.

Masters, William, and Virginia Johnson. 1966. *Human Sexual Response.* Boston: Little, Brown.

McElvaine, Robert. 1993. *The Great Depression: America, 1929–1941*. New York: Random House.

National Center for Health Statistics. 2001. *Births, Marriages, Divorces, and Deaths: Provisional Data, 2001*. Vol. 50 (14), 1–3.

Planned Parenthood Federation of America. 2001. *Pregnancy and Childbearing among U.S. Teens*. New York: Author.

Population Reference Bureau. 2000. *The World's Youth 2000*. Washington, DC: Author.

———. 2002a. *Family Planning Worldwide*. Washington, DC: Author.

———. 2002b. *Facing the HIV/AIDS Pandemic*. Washington, DC: Author.

Post, Emily. 1922. *Etiquette in Society, in Business, in Politics and at Home*. New York: Funk and Wagnalls.

Raines, Claire. 1997. *Beyond Generation X*. Menlo Park, CA: Crisp.

Reiss, Ira, and Albert Ellis. 2002. *At the Dawn of the Sexual Revolution: Reflections on a Dialogue*. Thousand Oaks, CA: Sage.

Sorensen, Robert. 1973. *Adolescent Sexuality in Contemporary America*. New York: World.

Thau, Richard D. 1997. *Generations Apart: Xers vs. Boomers vs. the Elderly*. New York: Prometheus.

U.S. Bureau of the Census. 2003. *Statistical Abstract of the United States* (122nd Ed.). Washington, DC: U.S. Government Printing Office.

Zemke, Ronald, Claire Raines, and Robert Filipczak. 2000. *Generations at Work: Managing the Clash of Veterans, Boomers, Xers, and Nexters in Your Workplace*. New York: AMACOM.

Zinn, Howard. 2002. *Postwar America: 1945–1971*. Chicago, IL: South End Park.

2

Issues, Controversies, and Solutions

We in the modern world live in an era of nearly overwhelming change, an age when the Internet has revolutionized communication and when palm pilots often organize people's busy lives. Today's adolescents are a testimony of just how much people's lives have been altered since the past century. They represent a new breed in a new age, and their differences are reflected in the way they act, dress, and even speak. Their many different dating activities create further distinctiveness, either with the new trends they've introduced or the variations they've spun on old themes: "clubbing," going to the mall, connecting on the web, taking in a movie or renting a video, watching the "tube," skating, shooting pool, or just "hanging out" or "chilling."

In studying teenagers' dating and sexual lives, one often comes face to face with an assortment of troubling issues, some posing a stark contrast to those of yesteryear, particularly in terms of parental concerns. For instance, whereas parents once worried that teens' sneaking a beer or two would tarnish their budding characters, the emergence of potentially lethal club drugs has produced new fears and apprehensions among parents. Along these same lines, although going to a movie years ago rarely prompted anyone to question the suitability of its contents, today, movie ratings need to be consulted before tickets are even purchased. And, whereas teens were once allowed to walk to and from social events because it was relatively safe to do so, this is hardly the case anymore. Indeed, in addition to arranging, or approving of, transportation for the evening, many parents insist that their teens carry a cell phone in their pockets and carry proper identification on a date, which for some means a *DNA Lifeprint card.* (The DNA Lifeprint card is designed to protect children from violence and other crimes. The child's DNA "fingerprint" is taken [the inside of the cheek is swabbed] and is preserved for more than fifty years.)

To be sure, the times have changed, and for better or worse, society is a lot more complex today than it was 100 years ago (or for that matter, ten years ago). Adjusting to change requires knowledge of change, and this chapter is designed to bring some of the more important and pressing issues to readers' attention. From this book's perspective, the demand has never been greater for people to better understand the following:

- Dating and sexual values
- Media impact on dating and sexuality
- Internet romance and sex
- Dating and club drugs
- Date rape
- Same-sex dating
- Premarital sex
- Birth control
- Teenage pregnancy
- Sexually transmitted diseases
- Cohabitation
- Teenage marriages
- Dating and sexuality education

As this book explores each of these topics, the theoretical will converge with the practical. This chapter will provide an overview of each issue or problem, including its scope and magnitude, the forces creating and shaping it, and possible solutions or interventions. This chapter also offers conjoined discussions of issues that are inherently related (e.g., premarital sex and birth control), distilling information that has been gathered from the vast amounts of dating and sexuality research that exist in the pertinent literature. A concerted effort has been made to apply the topics covered here to other chapters throughout the book, such as worldwide perspectives (chapter 3), notable historical events (chapter 4), and contributors to the field of dating and sexuality (chapter 5).

Dating and Sexual Values

There has never been a greater need for soundly held principles and values among adolescents, particularly in the face of such problems as teenage pregnancy, drug abuse, or sexually transmitted diseases. A *value* is what a person believes to be right or wrong, appropriate or inappropriate, or desirable or undesirable. Values related to dating and sexuality are important in shaping the overall lives of younger generations. Moral values are especially important—a person's individual ethical standards of right and wrong that guide that person's sexual decision making and overall standards of conduct. Such beliefs contribute to a dating and sexual value system that is unique to each person, a framework that enables individuals to appraise and understand their intimate relationships. In a broad sense, a dating and sexual value system represents a frame of reference, a set of principled beliefs that will shape an adolescent's involvement in intimate relationships.

In exploring important issues and problems in dating and sexuality, the topic of sexual values almost always heads the list. Although school systems invariably teach such values as citizenship and respect, exploring and discussing sexual values proves to be a more difficult chore (Despain and Converse, 2003; Scapp, 2002). Though most parents believe that the foundation for sexual values should be built at home, many admit to being uncomfortable around the topic or simply uninformed. If sexual values education is to be part of a school's curriculum, a number of questions often arise: For instance, when should sexual values education begin? Which values will be taught? Whose values? Will sexual values education for adolescents promote sexual experimentation?

Although more complete coverage of dating and sexuality education is covered later in this chapter, it is desirable to address the importance of these values early on. Dating and sexual values education is an important part of teenagers' overall schooling and will assist them when they need to make important decisions. Furthermore, values education is an important facet of character development, and as such, it embraces such virtues as compassion, commitment, and responsibility. When properly implemented and taught, dating and sexual values education exposes adolescents to the different values that exist and the practical implications of expressing them. In so doing, values education deepens teenagers' understanding, motivation, and responsibility with regard to their dating and sexual lives (Lickona, Boudreau, and Lickona, 2003; Lees, Muldoon, Sheehy, and Kremer, 2003).

It is generally recognized that the selection of dating and sexual values is a multifaceted process. Initially, individuals may be confronted with an issue that prompts them to form an opinion as to what is good or bad, right or wrong in that particular case. Examples of such issues are the acceptability or unacceptability of establishing an exclusive relationship ("going steady"), premarital intercourse, the notion of shared contraceptive responsibility, or the desirability of same-sex relationships. When individuals confront such issues, they usually recognize the need to establish some type of value for each one. Beyond consulting one's existing dating and sexual value system (which consists of the values that have already been taught), individuals may choose to solicit input from family, friends, teachers, or other socialization sources. The information and input gathered is then compared and contrasted, and one value is ultimately chosen (Lees, Muldoon, Sheehy and Kremer, 2003; Hutchinson, 2003).

Values may be extrinsic or intrinsic. *Extrinsic values* are derived from society's standards of right or wrong, which in turn are usually grounded in intellectual conviction. Because extrinsic values typically represent a conception of an ideal (such as values related to morality), they are sometimes limited in their practical application. *Intrinsic values*, on the other hand, are internalized from personal experience and represent those beliefs governing actual, everyday behavior. Because there may be a gap between extrinsic and intrinsic values, it is important to examine what a person says and how, in fact, he or she actually behaves (Scapp, 2002). For example, the person who acknowledges the importance of safer sex practices yet who still engages in unprotected intercourse reflects the kind of discrepancy that can exist between the two types of values (Lickona, Boudreau, and Lickona, 2003).

A number of social agents shape the formation of a person's dating and sexual values, including parents, siblings, peers, schools, religion, and the media. It is from such socialization agents that a *sexual value orientation* or standard emerges—an assumption about the purpose(s) of sexual activity and its place within an intimate relationship. Such orientations represent the basis for norms that specify what types of activity are appropriate and inappropriate and what types of persons are appropriate partners for sexual activity. The following are some of the more common sexual value orientations or standards that may offer guidelines for adolescents making decisions about their sexuality and sexual values:

Abstinence Orientation. This standard advocates the avoidance of sexual intercourse. Rather than sexual involvement, emphasis is placed on developing the romantic, companionate, and spiritual facets of a relationship.

Procreational Orientation. The procreational orientation emphasizes that sexual activity is acceptable only within marriage and for the purpose of having children. This orientation also views any behavior other than vaginal intercourse as undesirable.

Permissiveness with Affection Orientation. This standard views sexual activity as an extension of a meaningful intimate relationship. While sexual activity within casual relationships is considered wrong, sexual intercourse is viewed as acceptable if accompanied by love and emotional commitment between partners. Indeed, sexual intimacy within a committed relationship is perceived as enhancing emotional attachment.

Situational Orientation. The situational orientation suggests that sexual decision making should take place in the context of the particular situation and those involved. Rather than making decisions about sexual matters solely on the basis of rules, this case-by-case orientation carefully examines motivations and consequences. Thus, the acceptability or unacceptability of a sexual act is seen as depending on what it is intended to accomplish and its foreseeable consequences.

Double Standard Orientation. This orientation asserts that sexual promiscuity, particularly premarital sexual relations, is acceptable for men but not for women. Women are expected to remain abstinent until marriage, and, in general, to be sexually conservative. Those accepting this standard do not see men and women as equals, and they tend to align masculinity with such traits as power and control. Those rejecting the double standard often perceive it as being demeaning to women and lopsided in terms of relationship equity and balance.

Permissiveness without Affection Orientation. This standard, also called the hedonistic (pleasure-seeking) orientation, emphasizes the importance of sexual pleasure and satisfaction rather than moral constraint. Sexual desire is seen as a legitimate and appropriate appetite to be satisfied with maximum gratification and enjoyment. Unlike the permissiveness with affection orientation, which views sexual activity as acceptable provided there is attachment between partners, this orientation views intercourse by itself (without emotional commitment) as acceptable. Adherents thus see sexual gratification as an end in itself. Although society saw the hedonistic orientation being adopted by some during the sexual revolution, it is likely that only a small number of men and women live by this philosophy today. Fear of contracting HIV and other sexually transmitted diseases has created a shift toward more conservative sexual value orientations (Hyde and DeLamater, 2002; Crooks and Baur, 2001).

It is obvious from the foregoing that the complex and changing society of the United States offers divergent sexual value orientations, from abstinence to casual sex. Moreover, individuals are usually exposed to different orientations throughout the course of their lives, making value choices even more difficult (Ravitch and Viteritti, 2001). It should be pointed out, though, that these orientations are not entirely separate entities; rather, it is possible that some individuals incorporate portions of all these sexual orientations into their sexual value systems.

How might adults assist adolescents in their process of selecting suitable dating and sexual values, ones having intrinsic worth and validity to the individuals who hold them? This is no easy chore, as individuals must strike some kind of balance between what values they have been taught growing up and those that have become personally meaningful to them. Although the task here is not to evaluate dating and sexuality education in the schools, this book can share some advice and guidance. As stated earlier, the most effective values education for teenagers takes place against the backdrop of character development. To achieve this, many schools today are implementing character education coursework, seminars, and community service opportunities. *Character education* seeks to promote such positive standards of conduct as responsibility, respect, and caring.

Another point to keep in mind is that a sound value system and strong character do not happen overnight; on the contrary, these are processes that take time, dedication, and considerable deliberation. As they go through the process of deciding what their sexual values will be, teens need guidance about how to avoid making snap judgments that might cause them regrets later or gravitating toward specific values just because they seem popular or trendy. Here, as with other aspects of values clarification, teens benefit immensely from mentors and role models who supply information, direction, and advice (Despain and Converse, 2003; Crooks and Baur, 2001).

Once values have been examined and weighed, an adolescent needs to have faith and confidence in those he or she has selected. The overall system should be consistent with one's personality and everyday behavior; thus, there should not be a gap between what a person says and what that person does. Individuals with sound value systems also hold accurate pictures of reality. By this, they tend to be fully informed and up-to-date with their knowledge about dating issues and human sexuality (Crooks and Baur, 2001; Roffman, 2001).

Those with healthy value systems often recheck their values after forming them, testing them against their own subsequent feelings or life experiences. They are also tolerant of the value systems of others, being nonjudgmental and open to new ideas and suggestions. To illustrate, they are usually able to accept the sexual orientations and activities of others without feeling personally threatened or without moralizing or judging the other person. Sound and healthy values are also flexible ones, remaining fluid enough to allow for adjustment or correction. Finally, those with healthy value systems derive satisfaction from living by their chosen values—they provide meaning and a sense of purpose to one's life overall (Hyde and DeLamater, 2002; Lees, Muldoon, Sheehy, and Kremer, 2003; Hutchinson, 2003; Roffman, 2001).

Media Impact on Dating and Sexuality

The modern teenager is rarely away from the influence of the *media*, communication agents such as television, radio, and newspapers. For example, a television is available in nearly every home in the United States, and most teens have access to computers and the Internet either at home or at school. Other forms of the media are just as widespread, from magazines, movies, and video games to music and rock videos. The media are responsible for changing the landscape of adolescence and family life more than any other technological advancement of the twenty-first century.

A glance at some statistics illustrates how widespread media exposure is. On average, adolescents use media (all of the aforementioned types) about 40–45 hours per week. Adolescents watch television for about 15–20 of those weekly hours, and they listen to music for several hours each day (usually as background music or through headsets), which amounts to another 15–20 hours. Teenagers on average use the Internet about 10 hours per week, spending about 2 hours online at a time (Brown, 2002; Strasburger and Wilson, 2002; American Academy of Pediatrics, 2001).

These figures mean that the heaviest concentrations of activities for teenagers can almost be divided into thirds: 40–45 hours of media exposure, 35–50 hours of school (the range of hours is dependent on travel as well as on extracurricular activities), and 55–70 hours of sleep. To say that the media have become part of the American lifestyle is an understatement. Indeed, the manner in which the media and information technology have impacted younger generations in this globally interactive world has prompted some to call today's adolescents "cyber teens." This book's author tends to agree, so much so that this chapter includes a special section on computers and the Internet.

It is also important to note that many adolescents are sometimes home alone, often with unlimited and unsupervised access to the media. One study (Roberts, 2000) found that two-thirds of the teenagers surveyed had a television in their own bedrooms, many hooked up to cable and a videocassette recorder. And, even if parents are home, there is no guarantee that adolescents' viewing choices will be monitored, including the content of television, music videos, films, or the Internet. Research also indicates that with age, many adolescents begin watching adult programming, and usually watch it alone (Chapin, 2000).

Given such widespread exposure to the media, it is important to examine its implications for teen dating and sexuality. To be sure, mass media provide frequent portrayals of dating and sexual intimacy, and a number of experts (e.g., Villani, 2001; Chapin, 2000) have expressed concern regarding its content. More specifically, criticism has been directed toward media that either suggest or explicitly portray sex or sexual coercion or assault, drug use, violence, and other objectionable activities. Critics feel that such themes teach unacceptable behaviors, and they point out that younger generations are particularly vulnerable to the messages within such themes.

Such 1950s television sitcoms as *I Love Lucy* or *Ozzie and Harriet* hardly portrayed the characters as sexual beings at all, let alone addressing such topics as sexual promiscuity or unplanned pregnancy. In today's television programming, however, sexual content is commonplace, from daytime soap operas (which are quite popular with adolescents) to primetime broadcasts. *Music Television (MTV)* (a cable television channel featuring a format of music videos), and variations of it, constantly show teenagers a suggested sexual imagery as well as acts of aggressiveness, usually against women. Sex in advertising also exists both in print and nonprint form, as advertisers use sexually attractive models, nudity, and suggestive themes to build associations between sex and their products (Stern and Handel, 2001).

Fans of more traditional, family-oriented sitcoms are often hard pressed to describe today's television offerings. For example, a new kind of entertainment, *reality television* (a loosely scripted docudrama seeking to capture unfolding, real-life situations), has turned to dating for subject matter. Such dating programs (e.g., *ElimiDate*) have met with a wave of popularity. On such programs, a contestant is introduced to a pool of eligible dating partners. As the contestant dates each partner, cameras follow their activities and rituals, the centerpiece of which is almost always some form of sexual activity. Viewers, including teenagers, are given the message that character traits such as personality or kindness often take a back seat to physical beauty or sexual prowess. In between sexual escapades, audiences also see the world of material values presented by the media: vacation resorts, expensive meals, jewelry, designer clothes, and sleek automobiles. The program ends when the contestant selects the partner whom he or she enjoyed the most.

ElimiDate is only one of a wide assortment of reality television programs following the ups and downs of dating relationships and sexual provocation. For example, *Temptation Island* follows the exploits of couples who travel to a Caribbean paradise to see whether partners can resist the lure of infidelity and the temptations of bared bodies. Other programs deliver the sexual element in other questionable ways. For example, *Are You Hot?* gives contestants the chance to compete for the crown of the sexiest man or woman in the United States. According to the show's producers, talent, personality, and strategy are not required, just physical beauty and "innate sexiness." A mixed message is sent to viewers—especially teens—in a culture in which people try to maintain that looks aren't everything.

As far as the Internet is concerned, teenagers will discover that hard-core pornography is just a few keystrokes away. Victor Strasburger and Barbara Wilson (2002) tell us that such material ranges from lewd and obscene photographs to the Internet equivalent of "phone sex," sometimes with a live video connection. The transmission of illicit information via e-mail, or the targeting of children and teens on *computer bulletin boards* (which enable Internet users to post messages where other internet users can read and respond) by sexual predators, are other critical concerns. It is estimated that such websites and online activities have already generated billions of dollars in revenue, with even more predicted in the years to come. It is believed that half of the spending on the Internet is in pornographic enterprises. This topic will be revisited a bit later.

In addition to the sheer amount of media sex that adolescents absorb, concern is expressed over how sexual relationships are portrayed in these media. For instance, although promiscuous sexual activity has become a media staple, it is usually portrayed without reference to its risks and dangers, such as unintended pregnancy or contracting a sexually transmitted disease. Taking this a step further, Jane Brown (2002) writes that the media rarely depict the three Cs of responsible sexual behavior: Commitment, Contraceptives, and taking responsibility for Consequences. In addition, some intimate relationships are portrayed in the media with aggressive and even violent sexual content, as well as being influenced by the consumption of alcohol and drugs. Children and teenagers often have trouble discriminating between what they see in the media and what is real. Left unsupervised, as many are, younger people are often on their own to interpret the media's questionable sexual messages and themes.

Media images of masculinity and femininity are often distorted and misleading. Male characters are portrayed as being in charge at both work and play, clearly playing the protector and sexual aggressor in whatever relationships are at hand. Driving fast cars and often in search of fast women with reckless abandon, these rugged and strong men live a screen life of exaggerated freedom and independence. Even the number of actors in the media overshadows the number of actresses. In studies of television programming, male sexuality is featured more than female sexuality, often by a ratio of two to one (Chapin, 2000). Even the independent women who are shown on the screen frequently turn to men for directions or advice, lose control more often than their male counterparts, and become more emotionally involved (Strasburger and Wilson, 2002).

Media images of female sexuality also deserve consideration here, particularly the emphasis placed on physical attractiveness.

Adolescent viewers are led to believe that physical beauty and sexual attractiveness represent the gateway to self-worth, popularity, and success. The value placed on good looks is relentless and often succeeds in pushing women (and men) to seek an ideal of body perfection, often through surgical alteration. Because of the ideal body image being portrayed, many teens struggle with body shame. Sadly, media images of physical beauty are for the most part unattainable, because they have been airbrushed or have been altered by computer technology. Also, the emphasis placed on being slender or lean has led to chronic dieting, body dissatisfaction, and dangerous eating disorders such as anorexia nervosa or bulimia. *Anorexia nervosa* is a type of self-imposed starvation, and *bulimia* is gorging oneself with excessive amounts of food and then inducing vomiting or using excessive amounts of laxatives.

Liz Dittrich (2003) feels that the media often take images of thinness and link them to symbols of prestige, happiness, love, and success for women. Repeated exposure to the lean body shape via the various media can lead to the internalization of this ideal. It also renders these images achievable and real in the viewer's mind. Dittrich believes that until women are confronted with their own mirror images in the media, they will continue to measure themselves against an unattainable ideal.

In conclusion to this section, it is safe to say that the media greatly impact adolescents' perceptions and beliefs about dating and sexuality. Parents, and others in positions to motivate and guide young people, need to help adolescents realize that media images are often distorted and hardly representative of the real world. Teenagers must be helped to see that sex is not consequence-free and that lasting relationships are not more lust than love. On the contrary, teens must understand that relationships involve people, not sex objects, and intimate partner involvement requires love, commitment, and responsibility, not raging hormones and infidelity as often portrayed in the media.

Parents need to monitor the kinds of media being used by teenagers, and especially the sexual content of those media. The amounts of time adolescents spend watching television or surfing the Internet should be limited. Of course, parents need to serve as good role models by using television and other media appropriately. Parents also need to be knowledgeable about the effects the media have on younger generations, particularly those media having sexual content. Should media distortions of dating and sexuality occur, parents might want to use the program as a stepping-off point to initiate discussions about values, sexuality, and choices. Another positive step adults can take is supporting efforts to establish comprehensive media-education programs in schools; such programs often direct their energies toward critically exploring sexual content in the media (American Academy of Pediatrics, 2001; Brown, 2002).

Internet Romance and Sex

To say that the Internet has revolutionized the computer and communications world would be an understatement. Designed in the 1960s as a network to link university and government researchers, the Internet has become an information infrastructure that now spans the globe and allows people to electronically interact without regard for geographic location. Although originally a network of technical communications, the Internet today provides a variety of services and activities, including electronic commerce, information access, communication, and entertainment (Borgman, 2003; Gleick, 2003; Neville, 2002).

The growth of the Internet has been phenomenal. In 2002, it was estimated that almost 60 percent of the U.S. population (about 167 million people) used the Internet. New users of the Internet in the United States are increasing at a rate of more than 2 million per month. Worldwide, there are almost 550 million Internet users (U.S. Bureau of the Census, 2003b).

In 2002, the U.S. Department of Commerce released *A Nation Online: How Americans Are Expanding Their Use of the Internet*. This detailed and extensive government document provides a wealth of information regarding Internet usage in the United States. It is clear from this publication that younger generations are leading the way with Internet usage. In support of this, consider the following:

- Children and teenagers use computers and the Internet more than any other age group.
- Ninety percent of children between the ages of 5 and 17 (or 48 million young people) now use computers.
- Seventy-five percent of 14- to 17-year-olds and 65 percent of 10- to 13-year-olds use the Internet.
- Family households with children under the age of 18 are

more likely to access the Internet (62 percent) than family households with no children (53 percent) and than non-family households (35 percent).

- Households headed by single mothers with children under age 18 are increasing their Internet usage faster than any other type of household. Five years ago, about 15 percent of these households used the Internet; today, that percentage has tripled.

The most popular online activity is sending and receiving e-mail or instant messaging. *E-mail* is electronic mail, a message from one person to another sent by telecommunications via links between computers or terminals. An *instant message* allows users of the same service who are online at the same time to have immediate, one-on-one, private chats.

According to the U.S. Department of Commerce (2002), nearly half of the American population uses e-mail (45 percent, up from 35 percent in 2000). Searching for information also ranks high: approximately one-third of Americans use the Internet to search for product and service information (36 percent, up from 26 percent in 2000), and to search for news, weather, and sports information (33 percent, up from 19 percent in 2000). Figure 6.2 (chapter 6) displays the activities of Internet users.

By age 10, young people are more likely to use the Internet than adults at any age beyond 25. The high rate of use among children and young adults is reflected in higher rates of Internet connectivity within family households with children, as well as in high use rates among these age groups both at home and outside the home. In addition to schoolwork, children and teenagers also use the Internet for communication and entertainment. E-mail ranks a close second to schoolwork for the most common use for the Internet among teenagers and young adults. A high percentage of all teenagers (82.1 percent) between the ages of 14 and 17 and young adults in college (89.3 percent) use e-mail, compared to 45 percent of the overall United States population. These two age groups also go online in higher percentages than other age groups to engage in chat rooms and to listen to the radio or watch TV or movies. In chapter 6, figures 6.3 and 6.4 display Internet use among younger generations and the online activities they choose the most.

Without question, the Internet provides teenagers with a vast array of communication, information, and entertainment connections. However, it also has potential drawbacks: causing bickering among household members over computer time, interfering with teens' schoolwork, or detracting from family activities. Concern is often expressed that online activities such as games and chat are potentially addictive. Variations of these addictions can be compulsive web surfing or database searches, or obsessive online gambling and shopping.

Many researchers have directed their energies toward the Internet's delivery of sex and sexual content and the negative impact this has on young users (e.g., Cooper, 2002; Young, 2001). As we learned earlier, pornographic websites are widespread and are easily accessible by young and old alike. Cybersex addiction is not uncommon, such as the compulsive visiting of pornographic websites. Sexual predators also lurk online and attempt to sexually exploit children through the use of online services. Others seek to engage children and teens in sexually explicit conversations. Some predators collect and trade child pornography, and others are determined to meet youngsters in person through Internet contacts.

A recent study (Mitchell, Finkelhor, and Wolak, 2003) has shed interesting light on younger generations and exposure to Internet pornography. Surveying youths between the ages of 10 and 17, the researchers found that about 25 percent of the sample experienced unwanted exposure to sexual pictures on the Internet. The fact that the exposure was described as unwanted challenges the prevalent assumption that the problem is primarily about young people motivated to actively seek out pornography. Most of the respondents had no negative reactions to their unwanted exposure, but 25 percent of those who had a response said they were "very" or "extremely" upset. An earlier study (Mitchell, Finkelhor, and Wolak, 2001) reported similar findings in relation to unwanted sexual solicitation on the Internet. That is, about one-quarter of the solicited youths reported high levels of distress after solicitation incidents.

Finally, it was noted in the previous chapter that growing numbers of teenagers forge close relationships on the Internet, sometimes creating cyberspace romance. According to Sophia McDowell (2001), those who enter into such relationships are stereotyped by critics as being sexually deviant, highly reclusive, or relationally impaired. Opponents believe that computer dating promotes destructive and superficial sexual relationships. It is felt that such relationships place participants in harm's way for sexual exploitation, betrayal, and, should cyberspace partners be married, infidelity. Those who are more accepting of online relationships downplay these potential dangers, labeling such claims as simplistic and sensationalized characterizations of cyberspace interactions. Provided that participants are experienced with the Internet and the potential risks it poses, proponents argue that online relationships are an extension of our society's new age and the electronic ways in which modern people communicate. Whether Americans admit it or not, computer technology has become a mainstay in both our work and personal worlds (McDowell, 2001).

Regarding teenagers and online relationships, one study (Wolak, Mitchell, and Finkelhor, 2003) explored the characteristics of youths (ages 10–17) who had formed close relationships with people they met on the Internet. Females who had high levels of conflict with their parents or were highly troubled were more likely than other females to have close online relationships, as were males who had low levels of communication with their parents or were highly troubled compared to other males. The researchers noted that although little was known about the quality of the subjects' online relationships, troubled youths seemed more likely to be vulnerable to online exploitation and to other possible ill effects of online relationships. But, at the same time, it was recognized that online relationships might offer positive dimensions.

Given the amount of time teenagers spend online as well as their vulnerability, it is important for parents to guide them in some do's and don'ts of safe Internet relationships. To be sure, a number of researchers offer guidance on the dangers of troubled waters and how to cultivate healthy relationships (e.g., Clement and McClean, 2001; Fagan, 2001; Hogan, 2001; Adamse and Motta, 2000). More down-to-earth advice directed toward teenagers (e.g., Freeman-Longo, 2000; Aftab, 2000) details the hazards of online relationships and what safety measures must be practiced.

Certain themes cut through such publications, such as never giving out one's phone number, school name, or address, and limiting the amount of information shared with a partner. In fact, many believe that a red flag needs to be hoisted if there are too many questions being asked from the other end. Also, teens must remember that they never really know whom they're chatting with, nor what a partner's motives really are. There is much to lose by trusting someone whom one has never met in real life. Teenagers should never respond to suspicious messages, files, or pictures that are suggestive, obscene, belligerent, or harassing.

Also, teens should always be aware that *cyberspace stalking* can occur, which is unwelcome, unwanted, and repeated harassment and surveillance by another person on the Internet.

Guidance and advice about the Internet is also available to parents of adolescents, especially parents of younger teens. For example, the Federal Bureau of Investigation (2003) reminds Americans that many adolescents are moving away from the total control of their parents and seeking to establish new relationships outside their families. Although online contacts are to be expected, parents and adolescents should engage in ongoing dialogues about online victimization and exploitation. Keeping the computer in a common room in the house and maintaining parent access to online accounts is recommended, as is knowing where teenagers' other online activity takes place, such as at a friend's house or the library. Also, limiting Internet time in general and chat room time in particular is recommended, especially during the evening hours.

Dating and Club Drugs

One of the more popular dating activities enjoyed by teenagers and young adults are all-night dance parties, known as *raves* or *trances*. Although these parties offer young people the latest music and the company of like-minded peers (called ravers), they also expose teens to a significant health risk: club drugs. *Club drugs* are dangerous chemical substances that include Ecstasy, GHB, and Rohypnol. The popularity of these drugs—and the risks they pose—is evident in the following facts and figures:

- It is estimated that more than 8 million people have used MDMA (Ecstasy) at least once during their lifetime, representing about 3.6 percent of the population.
- In a 2002 nationwide survey of high school students, 7.4 percent used MDMA, 3.6 percent used methamphetamine, 2.6 percent used Ketamine, 1.6 percent used Rohypnol, and 1.5 percent used GHB at least once in the year prior to the study (National Criminal Justice Reference Service, 2003).
- In 2000, the U.S. Drug Enforcement Administration (DEA) seized more than 3 million MDMA tablets. This was three times the number of tablets seized in 1999.

- In 2001, approximately 7.2 million MDMA tablets were seized by the U.S. Customs Service. In 1997, the Customs Service seized 400,000 tablets.
- The number of arrests by the DEA for MDMA violations increased from 681 in 1999 to 1,456 in 2000 (National Criminal Justice Reference Service, 2003; U.S. Customs Service, 2001; U.S. Department of Justice, Drug Enforcement Administration, 2001).

According to Leshner (2001), many people think club drugs are harmless. However, they can produce a range of unwanted effects, including hallucinations, paranoia, amnesia, and, in some cases, death. When combined with alcohol, these drugs can be even more dangerous. Also, there are great differences among individuals in how they react to these substances. Some people have been known to have extreme, even fatal, reactions the first time they used club drugs.

Because some club drugs are colorless, tasteless, and odorless, they are relatively easy to slip into others' drinks. Some of these drugs have been associated with sexual assaults, and for that reason these are referred to as date rape drugs. *Date rape drugs* immobilize victims, impair their memory, and thus facilitate rape. Victims may not even be aware that they have ingested drugs or that they have been raped while under the influence of those drugs (Fitzgerald and Riley, 2000).

Given the many risks and dangers posed by club drugs, it is essential for adolescents and parents to familiarize themselves with these substances. To this end, the following descriptions of club drugs are provided by the National Institute on Drug Abuse (2002a). (It should be pointed out that club drugs are referred to by many different street names, and space prevents including all terms here. However, table 6.4 in chapter 6 provides a representative cross-section of street names.)

Methylenedioxymethamphetamine (MDMA). MDMA, known as Ecstasy or XTC, is similar to the stimulant amphetamine and the hallucinogen mescaline. It can produce both stimulant and psychedelic effects. Ecstasy is taken orally, usually in a tablet or a capsule. Ecstasy's effects last approximately 3–6 hours, though confusion, depression, sleep problems, anxiety, and paranoia have been reported to occur even weeks after the drug is taken. Ecstasy can be extremely dangerous in high doses. It can cause a marked increase in body temperature, leading to muscle breakdown and kidney and cardiovascular system failure. Ecstasy can also produce heart attacks, strokes, and seizures in some users. Beyond these health risks, hallucinations from club drugs can be fatal, especially if they lead users to engage in risk-taking behaviors or to inadvertently endanger or kill themselves.

Gamma-hydroxybutyrate (GHB). GHB, also called G or Liquid Ecstasy, can be produced in clear liquid, white powder, tablet, and capsule forms, and it is often used in combination with alcohol, making it even more dangerous. Many women and girls unfortunately discover that GHB has been used by perpetrators in date rapes. GHB is a central nervous system depressant that can relax or sedate the body. At higher doses, it can slow breathing and heart rate to dangerous levels. GHB's intoxicating effects begin 10 to 20 minutes after the drug is taken. The effects typically last up to 4 hours, depending on the dosage. At lower doses, GHB can relieve anxiety and produce relaxation; however, as the dose increases, the sedative effects may result in sleep and eventual coma or death. Overdose of GHB can occur rather quickly, and the signs are similar to those of overdoses with other sedatives: drowsiness, nausea, vomiting, headache, loss of consciousness and often short-term memory, loss of reflexes, impaired breathing, and, ultimately, death.

Ketamine. Ketamine, also called Special K or K, is an injectable anesthetic. When used in large doses, Ketamine causes reactions similar to those associated with use of phencyclidine (PCP), such as dream-like states and hallucinations. Ketamine is produced in liquid form, or as a white powder that is often snorted or smoked with marijuana or tobacco products. At higher doses, Ketamine can cause delirium, amnesia, impaired motor function, high blood pressure, depression, and potentially fatal respiratory problems. Low-dose intoxication from Ketamine results in impaired attention, learning ability, and memory.

Rohypnol. Rohypnol, or Roofies, is not approved for prescription use in the United States, but in Europe it is used as a treatment for insomnia, as a sedative, and as a presurgery anesthetic. Rohypnol is tasteless and odorless, and it dissolves easily in carbonated beverages. The sedative and toxic effects of Rohypnol are aggravated by concurrent use of alcohol. Even without alcohol, a dose of Rohypnol as small as 1 mg can impair a victim for 8 to 12 hours, which makes this another common date rape drug. Rohypnol is usually in pill form and taken orally, although there are reports that it can be ground up and snorted. Individuals may not remember events they experienced while under the effects of the drug. Other adverse effects associated with Rohypnol include decreased blood pressure, drowsiness, visual disturbances, dizziness, confusion, gastrointestinal disturbances, and urinary retention.

Methamphetamine. Methamphetamine, also called Speed or Crank, is a toxic, addictive stimulant that affects many areas of the central nervous system. Available in many forms, methamphetamine can be smoked, snorted, injected, or orally ingested. The drug is a white, odorless, bitter-tasting crystalline powder that easily dissolves in beverages. Its use is associated with serious health consequences, including memory loss, aggression, violence, psychotic behavior, and potential cardiac and neurological damage. Methamphetamine abusers typically display signs of agitation, excited speech, decreased appetite, and increased physical activity levels.

Lysergic Acid Diethylamide (LSD). LSD, widely known as Acid, is a hallucinogen. It induces abnormalities in sensory perceptions. The effects of LSD are unpredictable depending on the amount taken, on the surroundings in which the drug is used, and on the user's personality, mood, and expectations. LSD is typically taken by mouth. It is sold in tablet, capsule, and liquid forms as well as in pieces of blotter paper that have absorbed the drug. Typically, an LSD user feels the effects of the drug 30 to 90 minutes after taking it. The physical effects include dilated pupils, higher body temperature, increased heart rate and blood pressure, sweating, loss of appetite, sleeplessness, dry mouth, and tremors. LSD users report numbness, weakness, or trembling, and nausea is common. There are two long-term disorders associated with LSD: persistent psychosis and hallucinogen persisting perception disorder (which used to be called flashbacks).

What can be done to protect against club drugs? Education is certainly a step in the right direction, which includes building a foundation of knowledge, reviewing it, and applying it on a regular basis. Prevention is the best way to minimize the risks of becoming a victim of club drugs. As with other risks attached to dating and sexual behavior (e.g., date rape, sexually transmitted diseases), teenagers must recognize that the maintenance of well being is not automatic but rather is a matter of individual responsibility and intelligent and informed decision making. Research indicates that adolescents are increasingly aware of club drugs such as MDMA and their potential harm (National Institute on Drug Abuse, 2002b).

There are steps that women and girls can take to safeguard themselves against sexual predators who use drinks and drugs to incapacitate their victims. For example, it is important to watch one's drink (whether alcoholic or nonalcoholic) from the moment it's poured until it is finished to make sure no one slips a foreign substance into it (a designated and alert nondrinking friend is an added safety measure). Also, drinks should not be shared with someone else or accepted from a punch bowl or other common source. A woman should never let an unfamiliar man go off and get her a drink and bring it back to her. It is important to know the effects of the drugs and to take action if one starts to feel suddenly drowsy, faint, or unfocused. Should a person, upon waking up, discover signs that she may have been drugged and sexually assaulted, she should go the hospital immediately. Within a 12-hour window, the hospital will be able to test a victim's urine for GHB, which could make prosecuting the case easier (U.S. Food and Drug Administration, 2000).

Finally, parents must also frequently update their knowledge of club drugs and recognize that prevention strategies can save lives. Parents are the first line of defense against illegal drugs, and keeping tabs on teenagers' lives (where they're going, what they're doing, and with whom) enables parents to stay both involved and informed. Parents also need to realize that the raves where club drugs are used are often promoted as alcohol-free events, which gives parents a false sense of security that their teens will be safe. These parents are not aware that raves may actually be havens for the illicit sale and abuse of club drugs.

Adults should be aware of some other possible signs of drug use: because MDMA can cause users to involuntarily grind their teeth, ravers often chew on baby pacifiers or lollipops to offset this effect. Bottled water is often sold at raves, since Ecstasy causes dehydration in addition to its other effects. Ravers may use chemical "glow sticks" and flashing lights to heighten the hallucinogenic properties of MDMA and the visual distortions brought on by its use (National Institute on Drug Abuse, 2002a; National Criminal Justice Reference Service, 2003; U.S. Customs Service, 2001; U.S. Department of Justice, Drug Enforcement Administration, 2001).

Date Rape

Acts of sexual violence and assault are maladaptive behavioral responses, most always perpetrated by men against women. Rather than seeking sexual gratification, men who practice sexual coercion are seeking to control a woman by destroying her self-worth and dignity. At the very least, coercive sex violates the victim's rights. More often, though, it also brings degradation, humiliation, and a host of other debilitating psychological and emotional problems.

Broadly defined, *rape* is an act of a sexual nature that is forced upon an unwilling victim or that an unwilling victim is forced to perform on someone else. Approximately 300,000 rapes of women and girls occur annually, and about half of these rapes are committed by either an acquaintance or a friend. It should be pointed out that estimates on the prevalence of rape are misleading, because rape is one of the nation's most underreported crimes (U.S. Federal Bureau of Investigation, 2002; Tjaden and Thoennes, 2000a, 2000b).

Of particular concern in this discussion is date rape. *Date rape* is sexual assault that occurs in either serious or casual relationships. Serious relationships are ones in which the partners have known each other for some time, such as steady dates or perhaps former sexual partnerships. Casual dating couples might include those who have met at a party or on a blind date. Some may have met through a common activity, a mutual friend, as students in the same class, at work, or while traveling. Regardless of the circumstances, it is important to point out that date rape does not discriminate. It occurs in both heterosexual and same-sex relationships, and it affects victims of all racial backgrounds and economic situations (Fisher, Cullen, and Turner, 2000; Tjaden and Thoennes, 2000a, 2000b).

Although it is largely a hidden phenomenon because of its underreported nature, a clearer picture of this important issue has emerged because of the many female teens that have been courageous enough not only to explore their own negative experiences through psychotherapy and counseling, but also to confront their violators and to testify against them. This has enabled researchers to supply the public with important facts (e.g., Black and Weisz, 2003; Wilson and Klein, 2002; Chase, Treboux, and O'Leary, 2001). One of the more illuminating studies of high school students and date rape was undertaken by Jay Silverman et al. (2001). These researchers found that approximately one in five female high school students reported being physically or sexually abused by a dating partner. The violence that teenage girls experienced was strongly associated with such later problems as substance abuse, unhealthy weight control methods, pregnancy, depression, and attempts to commit suicide. Furthermore, victims were more likely to engage in sexual risk taking, such as having multiple partners or engaging in sexual intercourse without using a latex condom.

Like other kinds of sexual assault, date rape is an act of aggression and violence. More often than not, the rapist is seeking to assert anger, power, and control. Furthermore, men or boys who perpetrate abuse, violence, and sexual aggression are more apt to have observed or experienced abuse themselves. The National Center for Injury Prevention and Control (2003) sheds light on date rape with the following facts and statistics:

- Most female victims of date rape are between the ages of 12 and 18.
- Women and girls are more likely than men and boys to report being victims of dating violence.
- Date rate is particularly widespread among female college freshmen.
- Although victims of dating violence can be either gender, the injuries inflicted on males by females are usually motivated by defensive purposes.
- As the consumption of alcohol by either the victim or perpetrator increases, the rate of serious injuries associated with dating violence also increases.
- Several factors tend to be associated with sexual violence perpetrated by men, including the man's having sexually aggressive peers and the man's assumption of key roles in dating, such as initiating the date, absorbing the dating expenses, previous sexual intimacy with the victim, and a history of interpersonal aggression and violence.

The connection between dating violence and drinking is a strong one and cannot be overemphasized. Excessive amounts of alcohol have implications for the perpetrator as well as the victim. Many survivors of date rape report that they drank too much or took too many drugs to realize what was going on; by the time they realized their predicament, it was too late. Thus, the use of alcohol as well as other drugs impairs judgment and clouds rational thinking in dangerous ways (Wechsler, Fulghum, and Wuethrich, 2002). And, as noted in the previous section of this chapter, date rape drugs such as Rohypnol tend to immobilize the victim, making it easier for rapists to commit the crime. With a victim who is unable to resist and is feeling drunk or sleepy, the date rapist can take advantage of the situation. Such drugs can produce loss of consciousness and the inability to recall recent events. Some victims may not even be aware that they have ingested drugs or that they have been raped while under the influence of drugs (Fitzgerald and Riley, 2000).

Also, poor communication often contributes to date rape. For example, mixed signals may blur accurate communication. In one typical scenario, the woman acts in a friendly manner, but the man interprets this as an invitation to have sex. "No" is interpreted as "maybe," and even a strong protest can be ignored under the mistaken assumption that women say "no" when they mean "yes." Sometimes a woman is not clear in her own mind about what she wants, or she may think she will make up her mind as she goes along. Some men interpret a woman's nonverbal messages, such as her enjoyment of kissing and caressing, as meaning that she automatically wants to have intercourse. If she appears receptive and then changes her mind at some point and decides not to engage in sexual relations, the man may feel rejected and angry. At this point, he may decide he has been teased or misled and that he "deserves" sexual intimacy, regardless of the woman's wishes.

It should be acknowledged, too, that although date rape is usually a spontaneous act, many episodes are planned, some days in advance, others in the preceding hour(s). Sometimes a man plans to have sex with a woman even if he has to force the issue. These men have usually forced sex before and gotten away with it. They typically look for victims who are unassertive, perhaps someone who is not very popular and who he feels would be flattered to go on a date with him. Such men usually do not see themselves as sexual offenders. On the contrary, many are just out to enjoy themselves and have a good time.

Similar to other forms of rape, date rape has devastating effects for victims. The degree of trauma experienced is influenced by the circumstances surrounding the assault, especially such factors as the amount of violence, the length of time over which the assault took place, the type of activities, or characteristics of the rapist. Victims of date rape often experience shame, guilt, feelings of stupidity, and anger at themselves in addition to hatred, disgust, or anger directed at their attackers. Victims also tend to fear and mistrust men and even people in general. Many indicate that they have learned a lesson the hard way and are smarter and more careful because of the incident. Many also have difficulties in subsequent romantic relationships with other men, and they may tend to fear or be repelled by sex. Many try to block the event out of their minds and to forget what happened (National Women's Health Information Center, 2003; Russell and Bolen, 2000).

The long-term consequences for women who have been sexually abused or assaulted as a result of date rape must also be acknowledged. When negative attitudes about themselves persist, women may drop out of school or work. Worse, they may face life in general with reduced self-esteem. An important part of recovery is for women to restore order to their lifestyles and to reestablish a sense of control in their worlds. This can be a long process and can last from months to years. It is not uncommon for many victims to remain fearful or display other adjustment difficulties as much as one year after the assault. All of this implies that date rape has devastating effects on victims.

Experts agree that society must do everything it can to prevent this crime and to offer meaningful support and intervention to survivors. Regarding the former, the American College Health Association (2002) offers a number of suggestions to help reduce the risks of being victimized. For example, women should learn how to communicate their sexual limits clearly and firmly (e.g., saying "no" when one really means "no"). They also need to be aware that nonverbal actions or flirting may send unintended messages. Women also need to pay attention to what is happening and try to avoid vulnerability and dangerous situations. Finally, both men and women need to avoid excessive use of alcohol and drugs, particularly the health and safety risks posed by date rape drugs. For additional advice on sexual assault, see such resources as Petrak and Hedge (2002), and Riger, Frohmann, and Camacho (2002).

Before closing this particular section, it is important to briefly discuss the subject of stalking. *Stalking* is generally defined as unwelcome, malicious, and repeated harassment of another person, which causes that individual to feel emotional distress. Examples of stalking include following the victim, telephone or cyberspace harassment, sending unwanted gifts or messages to the victim, or surveillance. The latter type includes electronic stalking, which was mentioned in the previous section of this chapter. Stalking may escalate to physical assault, sexual assault, or even murder; hence its inclusion in this section of the chapter (Ramsey, 2000; Gross, 2000; Mullen, Pathe, and Purcell, 2000).

According to the National Center for Victims of Crime (2003), stalking is a gender-neutral crime, with both male and female perpetrators and victims. However, most stalkers are male. Stalking is not uncommon among teenagers, and it is particularly widespread among young adults. Stalkers come from every walk of life and every socioeconomic background. As far as motivation is concerned, some stalkers have developed an obsession or fixation on another person with whom they have no personal relationship (e.g., a movie star or professional athlete). The most common motivation, though, originates from some previous personal or romantic relationship that existed between the stalker and the victim before the obsession began (Pathe, 2002; Finch, 2002).

Stalking has many negative consequences, including many of the same damaging effects experienced by survivors of sexual assault. For example, many stalking victims fear for their safety and report exaggerated mistrust and suspicion of others. Others report anxiety, a curtailment of social activities, sleep disturbances, and depression. It is also not uncommon for stalking victims to have recurring thoughts about suicide. Because of the seriousness of stalking, all fifty states have enacted stalking laws. Although each state's stalking law differs in both definition and approach, virtually all proscribe behavior that constitutes a pattern of conduct seeking to harass and/or threaten the safety of another (National Center for Victims of Crime, 2003; Davis, 2001; U.S. Federal Bureau of Investigation, 2002).

Same-Sex Dating

Adolescence is a period of sexual awakening, and many gays and lesbians may decide to come out during these years. *Coming out* is an acceptance and disclosure of one's sexual preference. Some gays deny to themselves and others that they are attracted to members of their own sex. Others admit same-sex preferences to themselves, but not to heterosexuals around them. Such people typically lead double lives, enjoying same-sex contacts in secret and behaving heterosexually in public. But, some gays and lesbians choose to fully disclose their homosexual orientation, sometimes called "coming out of the closet."

Disclosure of one's alternative sexual orientation is a difficult decision for anyone, including teenagers. Indeed, to decide to come out may be one of the most painful yet important decisions a gay or lesbian person may make. Many communities in which people live and work are conservative in their attitudes toward gays, thus making the coming out decision even more uncomfortable for fear of repercussions.

Contrary to what was once thought, homosexuality is not a form of abnormal behavior or mental illness. Indeed, most gays are well adjusted and emotionally stable. Although some may exhibit anxiety or depression, so too do some heterosexuals. When maladaptive behavior does occur in lesbians and gays, it is more likely attributable to the social stigma attached to homosexuality instead of to something pathological in the nature of homosexuality itself. Additionally, gays are not inherently confused about their *gender identity* (the psychological awareness of being either male or female). Lesbian women are not any different from heterosexual women in their sureness of being female, nor do gay men differ from heterosexual men on this dimension.

Gay and lesbian adolescents can be faced with many problems stemming from others' disapproval of their sexual preference. They often do not feel as though they belong to any group and find they have few, if any, friends in whom they can confide. Although some colleges and universities have organizations for assistance and support for lesbians and gays, these organizations do not extend to the high school level because of legal concerns.

It is important to note that the problems encountered by gay or lesbian adolescents do not originate from sexual orientation per se. Rather, the problems stem from society's stigmatization of gays and lesbians. Rejection from family and friends, social isolation, and aggression from heterosexuals are problems often faced by gay and lesbian adolescents. Such antigay violence has risen dramatically in recent years. It has been found that many assailants tend to be white males in their teens and early twenties, who are acting out society's prejudices against gays. The purpose of the assaults is not theft, although this sometimes does happen. Instead, some people choose to attack gays simply because they do not approve of their lifestyles. Violence, intimidation, and humiliation are the means by which these attackers make their beliefs known (Stevenson and Cogan, 2003).

In the midst of such issues, experts recommend that adolescent gays and lesbians need supportive assistance and understanding. More specifically, programs emphasizing the physical, mental, emotional, and social well being of lesbian and gay youths need to be established. Staff development programs for professionals working with gay and lesbian youths also need to be developed. Also, gay and lesbian teenagers do not have many safe places in which to interact with each other in anything other than sexual situations. Gay and lesbian adolescents need opportunities for simple socializing, such as young people's social groups or dances (Berzon and Frank, 2001).

As far as the dynamics of same-sex relationships are concerned, more similarities than differences can be drawn between same-sex and heterosexual unions. Partners are sought so that a rewarding union may be formed, and the maintenance of a relationship hinges on mutual support, caring, love, and understanding. And, both straight and gay relationships tend to flourish when partners possess maturity and authenticity, a stable sense of self, and a willingness to share intimacy on a regular basis. For all people, the intimate relationship thrives on trust and commitment and offers such important social and psychological "vitamins" as security, affection, and comfort (Brehm et al., 2002).

However, there are some differences with gay and lesbian partners, including a tendency to maintain a more egalitarian relationship. For example, gay and lesbian couples are often free from the stereotypical form of role playing or mirroring of heterosexual roles that is sometimes attributed to gay couples. There is usually one personality that is more prominent or outgoing, but this "dominance" does not necessarily indicate that one partner plays the masculine, sometimes called "butch," role while the other assumes the submissive, or "femme," role. Indeed, there is probably more of an equality between partners in gay and lesbian relationships than in heterosexual relationships, because homosexuals are not forced into the types of roles to which many heterosexuals feel bound (Brehm et al., 2002).

Researchers have found that most gays want to have steady relationships, although this is somewhat more important to women than men. Heterosexuals, though, tend to value sexual exclusivity more strongly in a steady relationship. Both gay and heterosexual couples, though, desire certain elements in a close relationship: affection, companionship, and personal development. As far as qualities sought in partners, gays and heterosexuals both value such traits as honesty, affection, and warmth. Such findings shatter the myth that sex is the sole basis for gay and lesbian relationships (Kaminsky, 2003).

All of this means that gay and heterosexual couples are more alike than dissimilar in terms of relationship dynamics. Thus, if one wants to describe what goes on in a relationship between two gays—what makes for the success of that relationship and what may create problems—one does not have to use a different language; one can use the same terms as one would in describing a relationship between two heterosexuals. In people's intimate relationships, including during adolescence, we are all much more similar than we are different (Brehm et al., 2002; Clunis and Green, 2000).

Premarital Sex

Few topics about adolescent dating arouse more general interest and curiosity than premarital sexual behavior. This interest has led to a mixed bag of research findings, some seen as more positive and some as more negative. On the plus side, there have been significant declines over the past ten years in some very important adolescent sexuality problem areas: pregnancy, birth rates, and abortion rates. These declines indicate that more teenagers seem to be trying to prevent pregnancies, as well as taking a more cautious attitude toward sex. Also, fewer adolescents seem to be having sex, and among those who are, more appear to be using some method of birth control (Alan Guttmacher Institute, 2001; Annie E. Casey Foundation, 2002*).

Author's Note: The remainder of this chapter will be referring to some of the research originating from the Alan Guttmacher Institute and the Annie E. Casey Foundation. These two highly visible and respected organizations generate research and education in the fields of reproductive health and reproductive rights, with a special emphasis on adolescent sexuality. Alan Guttmacher was a distinguished obstetrician/gynecologist, author, and leader in reproductive rights. Annie Casey had a particular interest in providing assistance to disadvantaged children and teenagers, particularly those separated from their parents. James Casey, along with his siblings, named the foundation in his mother's honor.

The flip side is that despite such declines, the United States has the dubious distinction of still being among the world's leaders in teen pregnancies, births, and abortions. Moreover, sexually transmitted diseases in the United States, highest among adolescents and young adults, are higher than STD rates in other industrialized nations (Manlove et al., 2002). The next few sections of this chapter will examine these areas, the problems connected to them, and how to help adolescents create reproductive health behaviors that are more positive and beneficial to them.

Adolescence marks the beginning of the sexual and reproductive lives of boys and girls (see figure 6.5). According to the Alan Guttmacher Institute (2002; 2001), males experience their first intercourse at age 16.9, on average, and females at 17.4. Men spend slightly longer being sexually active before getting married: nearly 10 years, on average, compared with just under 8 years for women. By their late teenage years, at least three-quarters of all teens of both genders have had intercourse, and more than two-thirds of all sexually experienced teens have had two or more partners.

Levels of sexual activity and the age at which teenagers become sexually active do not vary considerably across comparable developed countries, such as Canada, Great Britain, France, Sweden, and the United States. However, problems such as teenage pregnancy do (see figure 6.6). Teenagers in the United States are more likely to have shorter and more sporadic sexual relationships than teenagers in Canada, France, Great Britain, and Sweden. As a result, American teens are more likely to have more than one partner in a given year than their international counterparts.

The Population Reference Bureau (2000) sheds additional light on international variations in adolescent sexuality and premarital sex. For example, in Kenya, there is more than a three-year gap between age at first intercourse and age at marriage; in Brazil, it is slightly more than two years. Around the globe, the onset of puberty is occurring earlier, which means that teens are facing a longer period of time during which they are sexually mature and may be sexually active before marriage. And, from an international perspective, it is important to point out that for too many young female adolescents, early sexual activity is not consensual. Children and teenagers are no strangers to sexual assault and coercion, whether in the United States or other nations.

Invariably around the world, premarital sex is more common among men than among women. In many communities both in the United States and abroad, sex is viewed as a sign of maturity and status for young men, but for young women it is frowned upon and considered shameful. This is a reflection of the double standard value orientation discussed earlier in this chapter. In the United States, many teens cling to this sexual value orientation. As a result, for many teens, traditional gender-role stereotypes may have been in operation since infancy, and during adolescence many males begin to act upon these stereotypes. Adolescent males are usually expected to have, and boast about (even if they don't "score"), sexual conquests. Adolescent males who do not experience premarital intercourse, or who don't want to, are often frowned upon by their peers.

Adolescent females, on the other hand, are expected to behave differently, at least according to the double standard. Many people believe that girls should appear interested in boys, but they should keep their virginity unless engaged to be married, or at the very least, going steady. Adolescent girls are often placed in a no-win situation. If they "give in" and have sexual intercourse, they are likely to be labeled "easy." If they hold out, they may be tagged "prudish" and not be asked out again.

A number of factors can be cited as contributing to Americans' high rates of teenage premarital sex. For example, much like other developed nations, the United States has become more sexually permissive. This book has previously discussed how growing numbers of adolescents believe in the relational or permissiveness with affection value orientation. This standard interprets premarital sex as acceptable, provided that it is accompanied by love and emotional commitment between partners. Also, as indicated above, many teenagers are also under strong peer group pressure to engage in sex. Experts on adolescent development (e.g., Cobb, 2003; Santrock, 2003) report that the desire to conform to the attitudes and behavior of friends is especially prominent among teenagers. Finally, this book has also discussed how the images of sex generated by the media are responsible, at least in part, for the increasing promiscuity among impressionable adolescents (Strasburger and Wilson, 2002).

It is important to acknowledge in this discussion, too, those reasons given by adolescents for *not* engaging in premarital intercourse. According to the National Campaign to Prevent Teen Pregnancy (2002), the primary reason among teens for abstaining from premarital sex is that intercourse violates one's religious or moral values. Other reasons for abstinence include a desire to avoid pregnancy, fear of contracting a sexually transmitted disease, and not having met the appropriate partner. One might point out, though, that although abstinence may preclude intercourse, this does not mean that sexual activity is nonexistent. Teens may engage in, say, kissing or fondling, but stop short of sexual intercourse.

The sexually active teenager is at a greater risk than sexually active adults for unintended pregnancy as well as for contracting a sexually transmitted disease. Serious risks and consequences accompany increased premarital sex, particularly when combined with inadequate information and inadequate access to reproductive health services. Also, unsafe abortion procedures can be added to the risks already mentioned. Sometimes, self-induced, unsafe abortions can result in severe illness, infertility, and death. Even in places where safe abortion services exist, access is often restricted for teenagers. In some countries, complications from unsafe abortion are the leading cause of death among teenagers (Population Reference Bureau, 2000).

This section closes now with an intriguing piece of research regarding when and where adolescents are choosing to have their first coital encounters. According to a team of investigators (Child Trends/Youth Risk Behavior Survey, 2003), although some adolescents experience their first sexual intercourse during after-school hours, the most common time period for this sample of teenagers (16–18 years old) was at nighttime (10 PM to 7 AM), with the most common locations being their family home or their partner's family home. Among those teens having experienced sexual intercourse, 42 percent reported "night" as the time they first had coitus, with an additional 28 percent reporting "evening" (6 PM to 10 PM) as the time. A total of about one-half of teens experienced their first sexual intercourse in their family home (22 percent) or their partner's family home (34 percent). However, young men were more likely than young women to report having intercourse for the first time at their own family home or a friend's home, and young women were more apt to report having had their first sexual experience in their partner's family home.

Birth Control

It was noted earlier that teenagers now seem to be trying to prevent pregnancies and engaging in better contraceptive use. However, given such high rates of premarital sex, coupled with alarmingly high pregnancy and sexually transmitted disease rates, much more improvement is needed. Too many sexually active teenagers do not consistently use reliable forms of birth control and do not exercise enough responsibility and rationality with respect to sexual decision making. Teens need a better understanding of those factors associated with sexual health and well being, including knowledge of birth control methods and how each one works (see table 6.5).

The lack of adequate contraceptive knowledge and use among teenagers represents a pressing social issue. According to Jennifer Manlove and her colleagues (2002), the lack of birth control must be addressed, along with other important facets of adolescent reproductive health: delaying sexual initiation, reducing the frequency of sexual activity, reducing the number of sexual partners, reducing the rate of unintended pregnancy and childbearing, as well as lowering the incidence of STDs. To do so requires taking a closer look at the range of factors that lead to positive reproductive health behaviors. Research consistently shows that teens who have information about reproductive health are more likely to use contraception than those without such information (Manlove et al., 2002; Planned Parenthood Federation of America, 2001; Terry and Manlove, 2000).

According to Jill Schwartz and Henry Gabelnick (2002), knowledge of contraception implies both thought and action. The person is aware of the accessibility of an available marketed product, as well as the products' acceptability and couples' willingness and ability to use it effectively. Contraceptive knowledge also embraces knowing a product's side effects and its potential failure rates. Methods of birth control must also be examined in terms of the degree to which they offer protection against sexually transmitted diseases. Knowledge of costs and the economic feasibility of a given contraceptive are important. Finally, what constitutes an ideal or suitable contraceptive method differs not only among individuals but also as individuals enter different life phases: a method that works for a sexually active female teenager who has had several partners, for example, may not continue to meet her needs as she becomes a monogamous career woman.

The Coalition for Teenage Pregnancy (2002) reports that contraceptive use among adolescents is inconsistent. Although the number of teens using contraception the first time they have sex is increasing, the number of teens who used contraception the last time they had sex is declining. Additionally, the following facts can help in better understanding contraceptive use during adolescence:

- There are approximately ten million girls and women aged 15–19 in the United States, 37 percent of whom are thought to be at risk for pregnancy.
- In their first coital experience, more than two-thirds of male and female adolescents rely on the condom. The older a teenager is at first intercourse, the more likely he or she is to use a contraceptive.
- The method teenage women use most frequently is the Pill, followed by the condom. About one in six teenage women who practice contraception combine two methods, primarily the condom and another method.
- Among male adolescents, condom use is likely to be highest at the beginning of a relationship, and then it declines as the relationship continues.
- The primary reasons why American teens have such high rates of pregnancy are less overall contraceptive use and less use of the Pill or other long-acting reversible hormonal methods, which have the highest effectiveness rates.
- The majority of unintended pregnancies among adolescent contraceptive users result from inconsistent or incorrect use (Alan Guttmacher Institute 2002; 2001; Planned Parenthood Federation of America, 2001; Henry J. Kaiser Family Foundation, 2002).

Unfortunately, there are often barriers that prevent adolescents from practicing effective contraceptive behavior. To illustrate, many teens find it difficult to obtain the birth control they need, because contraceptives are not provided in a manner that is accessible. Also, many parents shy away from discussing birth control or safer sex practices with their teens. Some prefer to remain silent about such topics, often assuming that their teens will learn what they need to know from school, books, or the media. Other parents believe that if they talk with teenagers about any aspect of sex, it will only serve to encourage sexual experimentation.

This latter notion, though, is not supported in the research. Indeed, parents who share a healthy relationship with their teenagers that includes honesty and effective communication are the ones most likely to instill sexual responsibility and safer sex practices. Further, parents who engage their teens in meaningful dialogues about contraception are more apt to promote positive reproductive health outcomes and fewer sexual risk-taking behaviors (Manlove et al., 2002).

Unfortunately, many adolescents do not use contraceptives or practice safer sex because they feel invulnerable to the risks of pregnancy or of contracting a sexually transmitted disease. Teenagers often think they are out of harm's way or are immune to the risks facing those around them. This is the sort of magical thinking in which very young children often also engage: "Nothing bad can happen to me." Younger teenagers, who may not yet have completed all the physical and neurological growth and development stages, may also have some remaining developmental limitations in their cognitive processes, which creates difficulty in fully understanding such issues as shared contraceptive responsibility, birth control alternatives, consequences of unsafe sexual practices, and perspective to envision pregnancy possibilities. Some teens, because their nervous systems are still in the normal process of development, may simply be too young to understand the needs of their sexual partners (including contraceptive needs), or to fully appreciate the notions of chance and probability attached to sexual risk taking.

Much has been made about this sense of invulnerability that encourages teens to engage in sexual risk-taking behaviors. Perhaps they need this seemingly impenetrable armor as they try to meet the many challenges that growing and maturing present. But perhaps, too, society can lessen this need with sexuality education that addresses such shortcomings in reasoning. The more society helps adolescents apply the information adults share with them, including realistically evaluating the consequences of sexual risk taking, the closer people come to bridging the gap between knowledge and action. The most effective sexuality education programs are those that help teenagers learn *how* to think for themselves, rather than telling them *what* to think.

Teenage Pregnancy

One would think that the 22 percent decline in teenage birth rates over the past ten years would be cause for celebration. After all, given the record high of 62.1 births per 1,000 females 15 to 19 years of age in 1991, the birth rate has tumbled to 45.3 births in 2001. However, the teen birth rate in the United States, although declining, still remains the highest in the industrialized nations. Particularly sobering is the fact that 40 percent of American women will experience pregnancy by the time they are 20 years old. Overall, there are more than one million pregnancies per year among adolescent females, and more than 500,000 choose to give birth to their babies (National Center for Health Statistics, 2002; Manlove et al., 2002; Planned Parenthood Federation of America, 2001; 1999).

More glaring statistics regarding this issue become apparent when one compares the teenage birth rate in the United States to those of other nations. Americans' teenage birth rate is more than double the rate for Canada, twice as high as England's, four times the rate for Germany, and fifteen times the rate for Japan. This country's high teenage birth rate places the nation in a grouping with Belarus, Bulgaria, Romania, and the Russian Federation (Alan Guttmacher Institute, 2001).

Declines in the United States' teenage birth rate have, however, been evident among all races. The most significant decline—21 percent—has occurred among African American teenagers, whose rate of births is now at its lowest in 40 years. Hispanic American adolescents now have the highest teenage birth rates. The following are some other facts related to adolescent pregnancies and births:

- About 13 percent of all births in the United States are to adolescent mothers.
- Almost 80 percent of adolescent pregnancies are unintended, accounting for one-quarter of all accidental pregnancies per year. Almost one-half of all nonmarital first births in the United States occur to adolescents.
- Fewer than 10 percent of babies born to unmarried teenagers are placed in adoptive homes.
- Most teenagers giving birth before 1980 were married, whereas most teens giving birth today are unmarried.
- Recent research reveals that, nationally, 22 percent of births are to teenagers ages 15–19 who already had a child (Centers for Disease Control and Prevention, 2002b; Annie E. Casey Foundation, 2002; Coalition for Teenage Pregnancy, 2002; Alan Guttmacher Institute, 2001; Planned Parenthood Federation of America, 2001).

Of the approximately one million adolescents who become pregnant annually, just over 30 percent have abortions. Much like pregnancy and birth rates, the abortion rate for teens has steadily declined over the past ten years. Adolescents currently account for about 19 percent of all abortions performed in the United States. African American females in general are more than three times as likely as white females to have an abortion, and Hispanic American females in general are two and one-half times as likely (Alan Guttmacher Institute, 2003; Centers for Disease Control and Prevention, 2002b).

Teenage mothers and their children face an assortment of health risks and disadvantages. For example, the younger the mother is, the greater the chances of infant death. It is estimated that the infant mortality rate for children born to teen mothers is about 50 percent higher than that for those born to women older than 20. Adolescent mothers are also more apt to have premature births than older mothers and are more likely to experience labor and delivery complications, including toxemia and anemia. Compared to women who delay childbearing, teen mothers are less likely to complete high school and more likely to rely on welfare (National Campaign to Prevent Teen Pregnancy, 2002; Manlove et al., 2002; Coalition for Teenage Pregnancy, 2002).

One source (Annie E. Casey Foundation, 2002) reports that about 75 percent of all unmarried teenage mothers go on welfare within 5 years of the birth of their first child. Additionally, about 64 percent of teen mothers in the study graduated from high school or earned a GED within 2 years after they would normally have graduated, compared with about 94 percent of teenagers who did not give birth. The failure to finish formal schooling can limit the mother's employment options and increase the likelihood that she and her family will be poor. And the roughly one-fifth of adolescent mothers who have more than one child are even more economically vulnerable.

The children of teenagers start out life at a distinct disadvantage. They are at a significantly increased risk of growing up without a father and of experiencing welfare dependency, poor school performance, insufficient health care, inadequate parenting, and abuse and neglect. Moreover, a cycle of poverty seems to follow the children of adolescent parents. They are more likely to do poorly in school, drop out, or become teenage parents themselves than those who were born when their parents were older. Finally, the problem of teenage pregnancy costs taxpayers huge sums of money each year: at least $7 billion annually in direct costs and lost tax revenues are associated with teen pregnancy and childbearing (National Campaign to Prevent Teen Pregnancy, 2002; Manlove et al., 2002).

Sexually Transmitted Diseases

Sexually transmitted diseases (STDs), sometimes called sexually transmitted infections (STIs), are contagious infections that, for the most part, are passed on by intimate sexual contacts with others. As many as twenty-five different types of sexually transmitted diseases exist; the major types are shown in chapter 6, table 6.1. Sexually transmitted diseases are quite widespread in the United States: about 15 million people are newly infected each year. Approximately one in four Americans will contract a sexually transmitted disease at some point in their lives (Centers for Disease Control and Prevention, 2002a, 2002b).

While the incidence rates of some sexually transmitted diseases, such as the bacterial infections syphilis and gonorrhea, have been decreasing over the past ten years, viral infections such as genital herpes and the human papilloma virus (HPV) have increased dramatically. It is estimated that 65 million people have contracted a viral disease other than HIV/AIDS. As far as HIV/AIDS is concerned, the cumulative number of HIV/AIDS cases in the United States in 2002 reached approximately 980,000. Worldwide, there are approximately 42 million people living with HIV/AIDS. In 2002, there were 5 million new HIV/AIDS infections worldwide and 3.1 million HIV/AIDS deaths (UNAIDS, 2003; UNAIDS/WHO, 2002; United Nations Children's Fund, 2002).

American teenagers are especially hard hit by STD infections. Of the 15 million new cases of STDs each year, about 25 percent occur among adolescents. Teenagers living in the United States have higher STD rates than adolescents in other developed nations such as England, Canada, Sweden, and France (Alan Guttmacher Institute, 2002, 2001; Centers for Disease Control and Prevention, 2002a, 2002b; 2001).

Infection rates of syphilis and gonorrhea are heavily concentrated among teens and young adults. The nation's most contagious bacterial STD—chlamydia—also infects adolescents disproportionately. Also, the hepatitis B virus (HBV), which is preventable with a vaccine, infects about 125,000 persons annually, teenagers and young adults being hit hardest. The human papilloma virus (HPV), one of the fastest-growing viral STDs in the United States today, is particularly prevalent among sexually active adolescent females. In fact, HPV infections of the vagina and cervix represent one of the leading STDs among female teenagers and young adults. Genital herpes is particularly widespread among older teenagers and young adults (Alan Guttmacher Institute, 2002; Planned Parenthood Federation of America, 2001; Centers for Disease Control and Prevention, 2002a, 2002b).

HIV/AIDS is also widespread among teenagers. Approximately one-quarter of all new HIV cases each year are persons between the ages of 13 and 21. The majority of these new infections are transmitted sexually. Worldwide, the situation is even worse. More than one-half of those newly infected with HIV in the world today are between 15 and 24 years old (United Nations Children's Fund, 2002; UNAIDS/WHO, 2002). In chapter 6, tables 6.6 through 6.9 provide HIV/AIDS statistics.

Why are adolescents in the United States so vulnerable to STD infections? Experts (e.g., Marks and Rothbart, 2003; Yancey, 2002; Hagen, 2001) point to early age of coital activity, inconsistent safer sex practices (e.g., not always using latex condoms), and greater numbers of both recent and lifetime sex partners. Males and females who have multiple partners over a specified period (e.g., several months) place themselves at increased risk for all STDs (Schwartz and Gabelnick, 2002). The use of alcohol and/or other chemicals by teens may also cloud or impair responsible sexual decision making (Wechsler, Fulghum, and Wuethrich, 2002). Also, because adolescents are less likely to be insured or to have a regular source of primary care, they are more likely to experience delays in the screening, diagnosis, and eventual treatment of STDs (Annie E. Casey Foundation, 2002; Manlove et al., 2002; Centers for Disease Control and Prevention, 2002c).

Female minority adolescents are particularly susceptible to STD infection. Regarding gender differences, all women have higher rates of infection from gonorrhea, syphilis, chlamydia, and genital herpes than men. Female teens also suffer more serious, long-term consequences from all STDs. For example, chlamydial infection is associated with the occurrence of pelvic inflammatory disease, which can cause infertility, ectopic (tubular) pregnancy, and fetal health complications. Female teens are also more likely than male teens to contract a sexually transmitted disease from any single sexual encounter. As an illustration, the risk of acquiring gonorrhea from a single coital encounter (in which one's partner is infectious) is about 25 percent for men and 60–75 percent for women. In 2002, women comprised 50 percent of the 42 million people living with AIDS worldwide (UNAIDS, 2003; Centers for Disease Control and Prevention, 2002a; Planned Parenthood Federation of America, 2001).

Minority adolescents have higher rates for sexually transmitted diseases, with rates for gonorrhea and chlamydia being substantially higher among African American and Latino adolescents and young adults as compared to their white counterparts. Rates of syphilis infection among African American women are more than three times greater than for white women, and the relative risk of death attributable to syphilis is also more than three times greater for African American women than for white women. Rates for chlamydia infection are also substantially higher among African American women as compared to white women. Also, HIV/AIDS takes a heavy toll on African American and Latina women. These two racial groups represent less than 25 percent of all women in the United States, yet they account for more than 75 percent of female cases of HIV/AIDS. HIV/AIDS is now the leading cause of death among African American men and women ages 25 to 44. It is the second leading cause of death among Latino men and Latina women ages 25 to 44 (U.S. Bureau of the Census, 2003; Centers for Disease Control and Prevention, 2002a, 2002b, 2002c).

Finally, the poor in urban areas are more vulnerable to STDs than individuals of higher socioeconomic status or those who live in suburban or rural areas. A number of reasons can be cited to explain why these population groups are more vulnerable: inadequate medical services, higher rates of other diseases, unsanitary conditions, overcrowding, and lack of knowledge regarding STDs as a whole. Among street and homeless teenagers who exchange sex for money or drugs, the risk of contracting an STD multiplies. Other groups—such as migrants and immigrants—may also be more at risk due to being medically underserved or difficult to reach through traditional health channels. Such groups may have language and cultural barriers to treatment and may also carry resistant strains of sexually transmitted diseases (Centers for Disease Control and Prevention, 2002a, 2002b, 2002c; 2001; Alan Guttmacher Institute, 2002; Annie E. Casey Foundation, 2002).

Living Together

As discussed in Chapter 1, cohabitation is a lifestyle status for couples who are unmarried, living in the same household, and who share certain obligations equivalent to a spousal-type relationship. Cohabitation is a popular lifestyle option for many people today, including older segments of the teenage and young adult population. Cohabitation has increased more than 700 percent since the 1970 census and has grown from 3.2 million couples in 1990 to 5.5 million in 2000. The majority of those living together in 2000 had partners of the opposite sex (4.9 million), but about 1 in 9 (roughly 594,000) had partners of the same sex. Of these same-sex, unmarried-partner households, about 301,000 had male partners, and about 293,000 had female partners. In 2000, California had more unmarried-partner households than any other state (Simmons and O'Connell, 2003). In chapter 6, table 6.10 displays statistics on married-couple and unmarried-partner households in the United States.

There are interesting racial and ethnic variations in cohabitation statistics. In 2000, about 17 percent of all American Indian, Alaska Native, or African American coupled households were unmarried-partner households. The Hispanic population recorded 12 percent of unmarried-partner households. The lowest cohabiting proportion, about 5 percent, was for households reporting a single race of Asian. About 13.7 percent of all cohabitants have partners of a different race (Simmons and O'Connell, 2003). For more information on racial and ethnic variations in cohabitation, see chapter 6, figure 6.7.

Many misconceptions surround cohabitation. For example, many people mistakenly believe that cohabitation is a lifestyle option chosen only by those sharing an intimate relationship, most notably those contemplating marriage. Although this is true for most, there are couples choosing to live together for purely economic reasons. Others may cohabit without any desire to become involved in a personal intimate relationship (Lauer and Lauer, 2004; Olson, 2003).

Other people falsely assume that cohabitation is primarily restricted to college students. Although many college students choose this lifestyle, so too do other adults. Regarding age variables, about 62 percent of cohabitants are under age 35, approximately 32 percent are 35 to 64 years old, and about 6 percent are

65 years of age or older. The average ages of cohabitants, many of whom will ultimately marry each other, is about 12 years younger than the average age of married couples. Nationwide, the average age of husbands is 49 years old, 2.4 years older than their wives. Cohabitants, though younger, are only slightly closer in age to their partners; on average, male partners were 36.8 years old, 2.1 years older than their female partners (Simmons and O'Connell, 2003).

One other myth is that cohabitation is chosen as an alternative to marriage. Although there are some couples choosing not to ever tie the knot, most cohabitants see marriage on the horizon. In this sense, cohabitation is a precursor to marriage, not an alternative. Before the sexual revolution, newlyweds took up a common residency only after their trip to the altar; today, many have already chosen a place to live and given it a trial run by the time they marry. For older couples that have been previously married to other partners, cohabitation could represent an alternative lifestyle to the one they previously experienced, especially if childbearing and child-rearing activities are not anticipated (Lauer and Lauer, 2004; DeGenova, 2002).

Given its popularity as a stepping stone to marriage, many researchers (Seecombe and Warner, 2003; Lamanna and Riedman, 2003; Cox, 2002) identify cohabitation as a transitional stage in the dating process: two people meet, date, fall in love, establish a mutually exclusive relationship, and then choose to live together. The increasing number of unmarried couples living together mirrors the more tolerant sexual attitudes ushered in by the sexual revolution (see chapter 1). More specifically, growing numbers of couples have adopted the permissiveness with affection value orientation discussed earlier in this chapter and see cohabitation as a natural extension of a serious, intimate relationship.

There are other reasons behind the popularity of cohabitation today. For example, in the college environment, such factors as the increasing availability of off-campus housing, coed residence halls, and liberal student attitudes deserve mention. Among all age groups, the stigma formerly attached to cohabitation (e.g., "living in sin") has lessened, while such values as individual choice and personal fulfillment have increased in importance. The popularity of cohabitation thus follows patterns evident among other developed nations, such as France and Sweden (see chapter 3). For those choosing permanent cohabitation over marriage, it may be that the perceived importance or status of marriage has changed. The same may be true for the perceived benefits of marriage. Adults who have witnessed their parents' marriages dissolving may have less faith in formal marriage as an institution that can provide security and happiness (Brehm et al., 2002; Olson, 2003).

As a lifestyle option, cohabitation has a number of perceived benefits. For instance, some partners enjoy this opportunity to combine love, work, and sexual intimacy in a setting that is free of parental control yet also free of the constraints posed by a legal bond. Also, for some, cohabiting fills a need to test their ability to relate intimately with a partner, a necessary skill for the survival of legal marriage. Cohabitation allows some couples to grow and change together without forcing them to make a permanent mutual commitment before they feel ready for one. And, it may allow them to separate without the burden of failure and guilt associated with divorce (Lamanna and Riedman, 2003; DeGenova, 2002).

But though cohabitation has positive features, it is not without its share of challenges. Potential legal problems are an important consideration, such as when issues of "rights" regarding property and earnings surface. Some partners report guilt over their living arrangements, and some are fearful of their parents' reaction to the arrangement. Because of the latter, many refuse to disclose their living arrangements to their parents. Another problem is that some cohabiting couples feel closed in and stunted by their lifestyle. It might also be pointed out that most researchers (e.g., Demmitt, 2003; Knox and Schacht, 2002) report that living together does not reduce a couple's risks for divorce if they eventually marry and that, for that matter, cohabiting is not always the way to a harmonious, stable relationship. Finally, unplanned pregnancy may complicate the lives of those choosing cohabitation over marriage. About 40 percent of couples living together have children (Simmons and O'Connell, 2003). In this scenario, should parents separate, the relationship dissolution can be just as difficult and distressing as any legal divorce.

Teenage Marriages

The vast number of family households in the United States consists of married couples, about 51.7 percent in 2000 (see figure 6.8 in chapter 6). For some teenagers, dating and courtship leads to marriage and they become part of this total, albeit a small percentage. For example, in 2000 about 4.5 percent of the nation's 15- to 19-year-olds were married. The United States Census Bureau uses this 15- to 19-year-old grouping in its reporting because these ages encompass the span of legally permissible adolescent marriages (Fields and Casper, 2001).

Interestingly, although 4.5 percent is a relatively small percentage, it represents a slight increase from previous years. The 891,000 married adolescents in 2000 represented an increase from the 598,000 in 1990, when married teens comprised 3.4 percent of all 15- to 19-year-olds. The increase came after a steady decline since 1950, when 9.5 percent of teens were married. In 2000, at least two-thirds of married adolescents lived apart from their spouses for various reasons; one spouse may have been in jail, away at college, or remaining in the couple's homeland. Research consistently reveals that females are more apt to marry in their teens than males (U.S. Bureau of the Census, 2003; Fields and Casper, 2001).

A number of factors contribute to the formation of adolescent marriages: a wish to accelerate the achievement of adult status, dissatisfaction with home life, loneliness, and the tendency to become involved in early and serious dating. For some, the threat of HIV/AIDS has encouraged a mutually monogamous relationship and perhaps hastened the ringing of wedding bells. Another factor could be that one or both partners are from nations where teen marriages are common, such as in Latin America or sub-Saharan Africa. Finally, couples in some states may have married to take advantage of programs established through the 1996 welfare program overhaul.

Pregnancy, however, is the most important factor contributing to adolescent marriages. Most teen marriages begin with a pregnancy. Eight out of ten babies born to married 15- to 17-year-old mothers were conceived before marriage. Each year, nearly one million teenage females become pregnant, which breaks down to about four out of every ten teenagers. But, as mentioned earlier in this chapter, the birth rate for adolescent females has declined steadily since 1991. To illustrate, the 2001 rate of 45.3 births per 1,000 females aged 15 to 19 is a record low and is substantially lower than the 1991 rate of 62.1 (National Center for Health Statistics, 2002).

Of the teenagers who marry, most are high school juniors or seniors. Many of the couples are not well educated and are of low socioeconomic status. Because their formal schooling is often interrupted, the occupational choice of married teens is frequently limited to unskilled or semiskilled work. Those who marry young also have one of the highest divorce rates in the nation. For example, in 2000, nearly half of the marriages in which the bride is 18 or younger ended in separation or divorce within 10 years. Duration of marriage is linked to a woman's age at first marriage; the older a woman is at first marriage, the longer that marriage is likely to last. In support of this is the fact that, for brides age 25 and older, only half as many marriages end in divorce when compared to teenage marriage dissolutions (National Center for Health Statistics, 2001).

Though some people may know stories of high school sweethearts who married as teenagers and lived happily ever after, such success stories tend to be the exception rather than the rule. Most teenage marriages are instead characterized by friction and an assortment of domestic pressures. For instance, marriage for adolescents tends to reduce partners' independence and autonomy. Researchers (e.g., Santrock, 2003; Steinberg, 2002) point out that adolescence is a life stage that supplies teenagers with an opportunity to explore and experiment, behaviors that greatly influence identity formation and other important personality dynamics. Marriage at early ages tends to reduce this freedom to explore, in the process curtailing important psychological growth (Cobb, 2003; Owens, 2002).

Financial problems also plague most adolescent marriages and frequently contribute to conflict and frustration. Many teenage mothers go on welfare within a few years of becoming a parent. For those teenagers who divorce, financial concerns are often cited as the primary cause of their marital dissolution. Although money does not guarantee marital happiness and satisfaction, a tight financial situation can create tensions and can aggravate existing domestic strife. One might add, too, that unemployment rates are higher among adolescents than among other age segments, posing additional domestic hardships and creating higher tension levels. In addition to disrupting family life, unemployment can have a negative effect on one's self-image and can lead to a loss of self-worth and perceived competencies.

The U.S. Department of Labor (2002a, 2002b) provides support for all of the statements in the foregoing paragraph. Younger workers are consistently more likely to be in poverty than are older workers. For example, among teenagers who have been in the labor force 27 weeks or more, 9.2 percent were in poverty, as were 8.7 percent of 20- to 24-year-olds. These rates were roughly double the rate for workers aged 35 to 44 (4.5 percent), and more than triple the rate for workers 45 to 54 years of age (2.7 percent). Teenagers must be helped to realize that education is of prime importance in getting a higher-paying job. Figure 6.9 in chapter 6 displays the projected percentage change in occupations based on the educational training required.

Finally, the introduction of children usually creates additional challenges for adolescent marriages. In addition to financial considerations and the further reduction of freedom, teenage mothers are more likely to give birth to premature and low birth weight babies. Mortality rates for both infants and mothers are higher during the teenage years. And, as mentioned earlier, children born to teenage mothers are more likely to be in poor health, be abused or neglected, and struggle in school (Children's Defense Fund, 2003).

All of this suggests that married teenagers—with or without children—are particularly vulnerable and require the attention of parents, educators, community welfare workers, and other social service agencies. Although the number of adolescent marriages in the United States is relatively small, they nevertheless represent a special contingent that needs continued social support and assistance (Mauldon, 2002).

Dating and Sexuality Education

As children and teenagers develop, parents and other caregivers hold them close for as long as possible. Their caregivers teach them how to take care of themselves and to be responsible. Their caregivers seek to transmit sound values and implant such important character traits as kindness, honesty, and respect. Caregivers, teachers, and other adults teach them important thinking skills that will hopefully enable them to always exercise good judgment. But at some point, caregivers must let go and have faith that what they have taught teens will give teens the ability to care for themselves.

But teens still need adults' assistance and guidance. Given the problems and issues presented in this chapter, it is critical for people of all ages to understand the thorny side to modern dating and sexuality: HIV/AIDS as well as other sexually transmitted diseases; epidemic rates of teenage pregnancy and abortion; sexual assault and stalking; club drug overdoses; and cybersex addiction. These problems have no easy cures. Society must work as a whole to help teens acquire a better understanding of the causes of such problems, learn more effective ways of preventing their occurrence, and find better ways for helping those involved.

Adults' dialogues with young people on these and other issues need to be age-appropriate, sensitive to teens' needs, and ongoing. Adults need to be open with teenagers and make themselves available to young people, and adults must be consistent in what they teach. The more adults young people have whom they can trust to share their concerns with, the safer they will be. Parents and/or other caregivers, as well as teachers, form a vital partnership and exert significant influences on a teens' dating and sexual behaviors.

Sexuality education begins in the home. During childhood and adolescence, young people are able to learn about affection, love, and relationships from those around them. Parents and/or other caregivers are instrumental in shaping attitudes, beliefs, and values about dating and sexuality, all of which requires comfort with the topics and good communication skills. A number of publications exist teaching parents and other caregivers how to upgrade their skills in these areas (e.g., Haffner, 2002, 2000; Roffman, 2001; Gordon and Gordon, 2000; Schwartz and Cappello, 2000). One of the chores facing adults is the need to overcome certain misconceptions about sexuality education. For example, many adults feel that if children or teenagers are interested about sex, they will always ask (they don't). Other parents and caregivers are fearful that providing information prematurely will lead to sexual experimentation and sexual risk taking. In terms of this latter myth, it has already been discussed in this book that meaningful sexual dialogues between parents and teenagers tend to do just the opposite: they encourage *fewer* sexual risk-taking behaviors (Manlove et al., 2002).

School sexuality programs provide opportunities for children and teenagers to become more comfortable with their sexual selves in many different ways. Effective education can teach communication skills, provide accurate sexual knowledge, explore attitudes and values, and address important sexuality issues such as those described in this chapter. Regarding dating relationships, education is often directed toward helping teenagers engage in responsible decision making and discovering the place of sexuality in human life and loving.

Unfortunately, not all schools offer such comprehensive dating and sexuality education. Instead, too many adolescents are exposed to presentations on only the basic reproductive facts—the "plumbing," so to speak, of human sexuality. Too many teens also receive scattered lessons from different sources that are often contradictory, less than accurate, or untimely (Somers and Gleason, 2001). All too often, sexuality education needs to sharpen its focus—that is, adults often devote their time and energy to coping with the aftermath of inadequate sex education: teen pregnancies, sexually transmitted diseases, and the like. In other words, society addresses teenage sexuality problems once they have occurred, but spends too little time helping adolescents to prevent the problems in the first place. Without proactive educational intervention, our society is creating sexually vulnerable citizens.

It is hard to understand why society has fallen so short in this area, when for years surveys have indicated that most Americans favor sex education in the public schools. As pointed out in the beginning of this book, perhaps it is because there is so much disagreement about the content of sexuality education, how and by whom it should be taught, and whose values should be conveyed. Perhaps some do not grasp the magnitude of the problems associated with teen sex, or maybe some feel that the problems will go away on their own. Regarding the latter, the United States has the rather dubious distinction of leading the Western industrialized nations in rates of teenage pregnancies, teenage births, abortion, and sexually transmitted diseases. The problems have not gone away.

When properly designed and taught, sexuality education becomes an integral force in teenagers' lives. It offers the opportunity to provide vital information, life skills, perspectives, responsible decision making, and insights that can make important differences in how young people feel about themselves and how they relate to their partners. The enjoyment of satisfying and mutually rewarding relationships should be a primary goal of dating and sexuality education. The best programs are those that connect sex education with dating and embrace such important areas as couple communication, commitment, values clarification, differences between liking and loving, and the importance of conflict resolution skills. Ideally, an effort is also made during such education to engage teenagers in the discussion and discovery of the highest possible character and morality ideals.

In order for all of this to take place, dating and sexuality education should place a particular emphasis on developing healthy thinking and reasoning skills. The topics contained in this chapter present compelling evidence that dating today presents numerous threats to adolescents' safety and well being. In order to remain safe, adolescents must learn to engage in thinking that enables them to exercise caution, carefully weigh risks, and not leave important decisions up to chance or circumstance. Moreover, sexuality educators need to emphasize instruction that bridges the gap between thinking and doing.

It has been previously stated that many teenagers see themselves as being somehow out of harm's way. This kind of thinking is called *perceived invulnerability*, a distortion of reality that sheds light on why teenagers are sometimes reckless or take unnecessary risks. Unfortunately, alcohol and chemical abuse, which tends to be widespread during adolescence, further clouds rational thinking and heightens risk-taking behaviors (Spirito, 2000). Adults must help those teens who engage in risky behavior; this is done by breaking the spell of invincibility they have created. To do this, adults need to recognize that this perceived invulnerability is often fueled by impulsive mental urges (e.g., "Whatever feels good, I'm going to do."). Adults must help teens downplay impulsivity and must teach them reflective skills, which tend to promote more systematic and deliberate thinking strategies and fewer unplanned and impetuous responses.

To reduce perceived invulnerability, adults also need to help adolescents better understand the concepts of chance and probability. Oftentimes, teenagers underestimate the risks they are exposing themselves to because they fail to consider elementary probability theory. More specifically, they underestimate the probability that their own risky behavior can lead to harm or injury. Sexuality education needs to focus on helping teens to better understand the relative degree of risk posed by their behavior, such as the chances of contracting a sexually transmitted disease during unprotected sex or the chance of experiencing negative side effects from club drugs. Put another way, teens need to realize that risky behaviors make them susceptible to more unhealthy or unfavorable consequences than they might have believed.

Other aspects of common adolescent thinking patterns deserve attention here. For instance, teenagers typically need assistance with perspective taking and with outgrowing the natural egocentrism (self-centeredness) of childhood, which often interferes with understanding the needs or viewpoints of others. Upgrading perspective-taking abilities and reducing self-centeredness pays dividends in many areas, such as better understanding the gender differences that exist in communication, appreciating the value differences of others, and engaging in shared decision making with one's partner. Heightened perspective-taking will usually blend with good communication skills to nurture such important relational components as mutual respect, empathy, and reciprocity. With such important psychological "vitamins" in place, dating relationships will likely flourish and endure.

Although thinking abilities, for most, develops in leaps and bounds during adolescence, it is important to remember that differences still exist. For example, some developing teens may still have difficulty separating fact from fiction, such as being able to recognize media distortions of sexual relationships or understanding why certain sexual behaviors put them at risk. And although certain information is usually understood easily, such as sexual anatomy and physiology, other topics (e.g., sexual values, self-disclosure, love) represent abstractions, and their many sides may not be so easily understood by younger (and still developing) minds.

This chapter closes by saying that, when done correctly, dating and sexuality education represents a true gift to teenagers, one that promotes responsibility and the ability to make informed choices. Sex education need not be the dreaded "birds and bees" talk by parents, nor the class to avoid in school. Instead, it should be a vehicle to promote healthy, safe relationships and a means to reduce the potential risks associated with sexual intimacy. Furthermore, the most important lessons to be learned transcend the subject matter and have invaluable life applications. That is, learning responsibility teaches teenagers that there are consequences attached to people's daily choices and that, one way or another, everyone is held accountable for their actions. Responsible choices are almost always informed choices, and responsible choices tend to breed such important character traits as confidence, competency, self-respect, and happiness.

Summary

The purpose of this chapter has been to present some of the most important issues and controversies in modern dating and sexuality. It began with a discussion of values, which are a person's individual beliefs about what sorts of dating and sexual behaviors are appropriate to engage in and under what circumstances. One's value system provides a frame of reference for appraising and making decisions about dating and sexual decisions. Examples of value systems include the abstinence, procreational, permissiveness with affection, situational, double standard, and permissiveness without affection value orientations.

Teenagers receive a steady diet of sexual images from the media in a number of different formats: television, the Internet, radio, magazines, films, video games, and music videos. A number of adolescent-development researchers have expressed concern regarding media content, including explicit portrayals of sex, as well as of sexual coercion, drug use, and other objectionable behaviors. Also, concern is expressed regarding distorted media images of masculinity, femininity, physical beauty, and general attractiveness. The relatively easy availability of pornography on the Internet lures many teens online, posing risks such as cybersex addiction and contact with online sex predators. In recent years, increasing numbers of teens have engaged in a phenomenon known as cyberspace romance. Although critics feel that cyberspace romance has a tendency to promote superficial, destructive relationships, proponents see it as an extension of modern life and a meaningful way to connect in the modern electronic world.

Should their dating activities consist of all-night dance parties, or "raves," adolescents may be exposed to club drugs, a class of dangerous substances including Ecstasy, GHB, and Rohypnol. Club drugs produce a wide range of unwanted effects, and some have been associated with date rape, a type of sexual assault that can occur in both casual and serious relationships. Although date rape is widespread among adolescents, it is an underreported crime, and experts agree that society must do everything possible to offer meaningful support and intervention. Another danger is stalking, which can escalate to sexual assault. Stalking is the unwelcome, malicious, and repeated harassment of another person.

It is during adolescence that many gays and lesbians engage in coming out, an acceptance and disclosure of their sexual preference. Though homosexuality is not a form of abnormal behavior or mental illness, many adolescents are faced with problems originating from society's disapproval of their sexual preference. Same-sex relationships are more alike than dissimilar to heterosexual unions. In both types of relationships, partners are sought so that a rewarding union may be formed, and the maintenance of the relationship hinges on mutual support, caring, love, and understanding.

By the end of adolescence, most teenagers of both genders have experienced sexual intercourse, and more than two-thirds of all sexually experienced teenagers have had two or more partners. Although levels of sexual activity among American teenagers do not vary considerably from those of comparable developed nations, the problems accompanying American adolescents' sexual activity do vary from those of other nations. Despite significant declines over the past 10 years in rates of teenage pregnancy, birth, and abortion, the United States still leads industrialized nations in these problem areas. Furthermore, rates of STD infection are higher in the United States than the rates in other industrialized nations.

Many older adolescents and young adults choose to live together in an unmarried relationship, known as cohabitation. Cohabitation has sharply increased over the past thirty years, prompting many researchers to include it as a stage of the dating process. Contrary to what many people think, cohabitation is not usually chosen as an alternative to marriage. The percentage of marriages involving teenagers is small, although a slight increase has been reported over the past few years. Many teenage marriages are beset with adjustment difficulties, often accentuated by financial hardship, low educational attainment, and the additional stress of raising children. Adolescent marriages have one of the highest divorce rates in the nation.

The chapter ended with some food for thought regarding dating and sexuality education. At the very least, dating and sexuality education must tackle the tough issues currently making the headlines—inappropriately high rates of teenage pregnancy, birth, abortion, and sexually transmitted diseases. A proactive approach that emphasizes the twin forces of knowledge and prevention is needed, with a particular emphasis placed on changing adolescents' thinking patterns, some of which may often be left over from earlier developmental stages of life. Adolescents' frequently held notion of perceived invulnerability is a thread that winds its way through most of the problems discussed in this chapter, and intervention must find ways to somehow break this spell of invincibility. Only then will teenagers be truly able to understand how fragile life can be and how people's values and choices must be guided by clear thinking and sound decision making.

References

Adamse, Michael, and Sheree Motta. 2000. *Affairs of the Net: The Cybershrinks' Guide to Online Relationships.* Deerfield Beach, FL: Health Communications.

Aftab, Parry. 2000. *The Parent's Guide to Protecting Your Children in Cyberspace.* New York: McGraw-Hill.

Alan Guttmacher Institute. 2001. *Teenagers' Sexual and Reproductive Health.* New York: Author.

———. 2002. *Sexual and Reproductive Health of Women and Men.* New York: Author.

———. 2003. *Induced Abortion: Fact Sheet.* New York: Author.

American Academy of Pediatrics. 2001. "Sexuality, Contraception, and the Media." *Pediatrics,* 107 (1), 11–19.

American College Health Association. 2002. *Acquaintance Rape: What Everyone Should Know.* Baltimore, MD: ACHA.

Annie E. Casey Foundation. 2002. *2002 Kids Count Data Book.* Baltimore, MD: Author.

Berzon, Betty, and Barney Frank (Eds.). 2001. *Positively Gay: New Approaches to Gay and Lesbian Life.* Berkeley, CA: Ten Speed.

Black, Barbara, and Maureen Weisz. 2003. "Dating Violence: Help-Seeking Behaviors of African American Middle Schoolers." *Violence against Women,* 9 (2), 187–206.

Borgman, Christine. 2003. *From Gutenberg to the Global Information Infrastructure: Access to Information in the Networked World.* Cambridge, MA: MIT Press.

Brehm, Sharon, Rowland S. Miller, Daniel Perlman, and Susan Campbell. 2002. *Intimate Relationships (3rd Ed.).* New York: McGraw-Hill.

Brown, Jane D. 2002. "Mass Media Influences on Sexuality." *Journal of Sex Research,* 39 (1), 5–13.

Centers for Disease Control and Prevention. 2001. *Tracking the Hidden Epidemics: Trends in STDs in the United States.* Atlanta, GA: Author.

Centers for Disease Control and Prevention. 2002a. National Center for HIV, STD, and TB Prevention. *HIV/AIDS Surveillance Report.* Atlanta, GA: Author.

Centers for Disease Control and Prevention. 2002b. Trends in Sexual Risk Behaviors among High School Students—United States, 1991–2001. *Morbidity and Mortality Weekly Report,* 51 (38), 856–859.

Centers for Disease Control and Prevention. 2002c. *Sexually Transmitted Diseases Treatment Guidelines.* Atlanta, GA: Author.

Chapin, John R. 2000. "Adolescent Sex and the Mass Media: A Developmental Approach." *Adolescence,* 35 (14), 140–151.

Chase, Kenneth, Dominique Treboux, and K. Daniel O'Leary. 2001. "Characteristics of High-Risk Adolescents' Dating Violence." *Journal of Interpersonal Violence,* 17 (1), 33–49.

Child Trends/Youth Risk Behavior Survey. 2003. *Facts at a Glance* (Winter). Washington, DC: Child Trends.

Children's Defense Fund. 2003. *The State of Children in America's Union 2002.* Washington, DC: Author.

Clement, Christy, and Kay McClean. 2001. *Wired, Not Weird: A Woman's Guide to Dating Online.* Annadale, VA: Synergy.

Clunis, M., and G. Dorsey Green. 2000. *Lesbian Couples: A Guide to Creating Healthy Relationships.* New York: Avalon.

Coalition for Teenage Pregnancy. 2002. *Recent Trends in Teen Pregnancy, Sexual Activity, and Contraceptive Use.* Washington, DC: Author.

Cobb, Nancy. 2003. *Adolescence (5th Ed.).* New York: McGraw-Hill.

Cooper, Albert. 2002. *Sex and the Internet: A Guide Book for Clinicians.* Bristol, PA: Taylor and Francis.

Cox, Frank. 2002. *Human Intimacy: Marriage, the Family and its Meaning.* Fresno, CA: Thomson.

Crooks, Robert L., and Karla Baur. 2001. *Our Sexuality.* Monterey, CA: Wadsworth.

Davis, Joseph A. 2001. *Stalking Crimes and Victim Protection: Prevention, Intervention, Threat Assessment, and Civil Management.* Boca Raton, FL: CRC Press.

DeGenova, Mary Kay. 2002. *Intimate Relationships, Marriages and Families (5th Ed.).* New York: McGraw-Hill.

Demmitt, Kevin. 2003. *Marriage and Family.* Fresno, CA: Thomson.

Despain, James, and Jane B. Converse. 2003. *And Dignity for All: Unlocking Greatness with Values-Based Leadership.* Dallas, TX: Pearson Educational.

Dittrich, Liz. 2003. *About Face Facts on the Media.* Retrieved January 22, 2003, from: http://www.about-face.org/r/facts/media.html.

Fagan, Eric. 2001. *Cast Your Net: A Step-By-Step Guide for Finding Your Soulmate on the Internet.* New York: Harvard Common Press.

Federal Bureau of Investigation. 2003. *A Parent's Guide to Internet Safety.* Retrieved March 29, 2003, from: http://www.fbi.gov/publications/pguide/pguidee.htm.

Fields, Jason, and Lynne M. Casper. 2001. *Current Population Reports.* Washington, DC: U.S. Census Bureau, Department of Commerce, June.

Finch, Emily. 2002. *The Criminalization of Stalking: Constructing the Problem and Evaluating the Solution.* London: Cavendish.

Fisher, Bonnie S., Francis T. Cullen, and Michael G. Turner. 2000. *Sexual Victimization of College Women.* Washington, DC: U.S. Department of Justice, National Institute of Justice.

Fitzgerald, Nora, and K. Jack Riley. 2000. "Drug-Facilitated Rape: Looking for the Missing Pieces." *National Institute of Justice Journal,* 14 (4), 8–15.

Freeman-Longo, Richard E. 2000. "Children, Teens and Sex on the Internet." *Sexual Addiction & Compulsivity, 7,* 75–90.

Gleick, James. 2003. *What Just Happened: A Chronicle from the Information Frontier.* New York: Vintage.

Gordon, Sol, and Judith Gordon. 2000. *Raising a Child Responsibly in a Sexually Permissive World.* Holbrook, MA: Adams Media.

Gross, Linden. 2000. *Surviving a Stalker: Everything You Need to Know to Keep Yourself Safe.* New York: Marlowe.

Haffner, Debra W. 2000. *From Diapers to Dating: A Parent's Guide to Raising Sexually Healthy Children.* New York: Newmarket.

———. 2002. *Beyond the Big Talk: Every Parent's Guide to Raising Sexually Healthy Teens, from Middle School to High School and Beyond.* New York: Newmarket.

Hagen, Ronald. 2001. *STDs: What You Don't Know Can Hurt You.* New York: iUniverse.

Henry J. Kaiser Family Foundation. 2002. *Contraceptive Use and Methods in the United States.* Menlo Park, CA: Author.

Hogan, Eve E. 2001. *Virtual Foreplay: Making Your Online Relationship a Real-Life Success.* Emeryville, CA: Hunter House.

Hutchinson, Elizabeth. 2003. *Dimensions of Human Behavior.* Thousand Oaks, CA: Sage.

Hyde, Janet S. and John DeLamater. 2002. *Understanding Human Sexuality.* New York: McGraw-Hill.

Kaminsky, Neil. 2003. *Affirmative Gay Relationships.* Binghamton, NY: Haworth.

Knox, David, and Caroline Schacht. 2002. *Choices in Relationships: An Introduction to Marriage and the Family.* Fresno, CA: Thomson.

Lamanna, Mary Ann, and Agnes Riedman. 2003. *Marriages and Families: Making Choices in a Diverse Society.* Fresno, CA: Thomson.

Lauer, Robert, and Jeanette C. Lauer. In press. *Marriage and Family (5th Ed.).* New York: McGraw-Hill.

Lees, Stanley, Orla Muldoon, Noel Sheehy, and John Kremer. (Eds.). 2003. *Applying Social Psychology.* Indianapolis, IN: Macmillan.

Leshner, Alan I. 2001. "Club Drugs Aren't "'Fun Drugs.'" National Institute on Drug Abuse. Retrieved March 29, 2003, from: http://www.drugabuse. gov/Published_Articles/fundrugs.html.

Lickona, Thomas, William Boudreau, and Judy Lickona. 2003. *Sex, Love and You: Making the Right Decision.* South Bend, IN: Ave Maria.

Mancilla, Michael, and Lisa Troshinsky. 2003. *Love in the Time of HIV: The Gay Man's Guide to Sex, Dating, and Relationships.* New York: Guilford Press.

Manlove, Jennifer, Elizabeth Terry-Humen, Angela R. Papillo, Kerry Franzetta, Stephanie Williams, and Suzanne Ryan. 2002. *Preventing Teenage Pregnancy, Childbearing, and Sexually Transmitted Diseases: What the Research Shows.* Washington, DC: Child Trends.

Marks, Andrea, and Betty Rothbart. 2003. *Healthy Teens, Body and Soul: A Parent's Complete Guide to Adolescent Health.* New York: Simon and Schuster.

Mauldon, Jane. 2002. "Families Started by Teenagers." In Mary Ann Mason, Arlene Skolnick, and Stephen D. Sugarman (Eds.). *All Our Families: New Policies for a New Century (2nd Ed.).* Cary, NC: Oxford University Press.

McDowell, Sophia W. 2001. *The Development of Online and Offline Romantic Relationships: A Turning Point Study.* Retrieved March 29, 2003, from: http://www.internetromance.org/thesis.htm.

Mitchell, Kimberly, David Finkelhor, and Janis Wolak. 2001. "Risk Factors for and Impact of Online Solicitation of Youth." *Journal of the American Medical Association,* 285 (23): 3011–3014.

———. 2003. "The Exposure of Youth to Unwanted Sexual Material on the Internet: A National Survey of Risk, Impact and Prevention." *Youth & Society,* 34 (3): 330–358.

Mullen, Paul E., Michele Pathe, and Rosemary Purcell. 2000. *Stalkers and Their Victims.* Port Chester, NY: Cambridge University Press.

National Campaign to Prevent Teen Pregnancy. 2002. *Fact Sheet: Recent Trends in Teen Pregnancy, Sexual Activity, and Contraceptive Use.* Washington, DC: Author.

National Center for Health Statistics. 2001. *First Marriage Dissolution, Divorce, and Remarriage: United States.* Hyattsville, MD: U.S. Department of Health and Human Services.

————. 2002. *Teenage Births in the United States.* Hyattsville, MD: U.S. Department of Health and Human Services.

National Center for Injury Prevention and Control. 2003. *Dating Violence.* Atlanta, GA: Centers for Disease Control and Prevention.

National Center for Victims of Crime. 2003. *Stalking Resource Center Newsletter* (Winter). Washington, DC: U.S. Department of Justice.

National Criminal Justice Reference Service. 2003. *Club Drugs: Facts and Figures.* Retrieved March 29, 2003, from: http://www.ncjrs.org/club_drugs/facts.html.

National Institute on Drug Abuse. 2002a. *Club Drugs.* Retrieved March 29, 2003, from: http://165.112.78.61/ClubAlert/ClubdrugAlert.html.

————. 2002b. *Monitoring the Future: A Continuing Study of American Youth.* Retrieved March 6, 2003, from: http://www.drugabuse.gov/Newsroom/02/NR12–16.html.

National Women's Health Information Center. 2003. *Violence against Women.* Washington, DC: Department of Health and Human Services.

Neville, Kristine. 2002. *Communicate and Connect to the Internet.* New York: Gateway.

Olson, David. 2003. *Marriages and Families: Intimacy, Diversity and Strengths (4th Ed.).* New York: McGraw-Hill.

Owens, Karen B. 2002. *Child and Adolescent Development: An Integrated Approach.* Fresno, CA: Thomson.

Pathe, Michele. 2002. *Surviving Stalking.* Port Chester, NY: Cambridge University Press.

Petrak, Jenny, and Barbara Hedge. 2002. *Trauma of Sexual Assault: Treatment, Prevention and Practice.* New York: Wiley.

Planned Parenthood Federation of America. 1999. *Fact Sheet: Pregnancy and Childbearing among United States Teenagers.* New York: Author.

————. 2001. *White Paper: Adolescent Sexuality.* New York: Author.

Population Reference Bureau. 2000. *The World's Youth 2000.* Washington, DC: Author.

Ramsey, Betsy. 2000. *Stop the Stalker: A Guide for Targets*. Morrow, GA: Securus House.

Ravitch, Diane, and Joseph Viteritti. 2001. *Making Good Citizens*. New Haven, CT: Yale University Press.

Riger, Stephanie, Lisa Frohmann, and Jennifer Camacho. 2002. *Evaluating Services for Survivors of Domestic Violence and Sexual Assault*. Thousand Oaks, CA: Sage.

Roberts, Donald F. 2000. "Media and Youth: Access, Exposure and Privatization." *Journal of Adolescent Health*, 27 (2): 8–14.

Roffman, Deborah M. 2001. *Sex and Sensibility: The Thinking Parent's Guide to Talking Sense about Sex*. Scranton, PA: Perseus.

Russell, Diana E., and Rebecca M. Bolen. 2000. *The Epidemic of Rape and Child Sexual Abuse in the United States*. Thousand Oaks, CA: Sage.

Santrock, John W. 2003. *Adolescence (9th Ed.)*. New York: McGraw-Hill.

Scapp, Ronald. 2002. *Teaching Values: Education, Politics and Culture*. Florence, KY: Routledge.

Schwartz, Jill L., and Henry L. Gabelnick. 2002. "Current Contraceptive Research." *Perspectives on Sexual and Reproductive Health*, 34 (6): 11–17.

Schwartz, Pepper, and Dominic Cappello. 2000. *Ten Talks Parents Must Have with Their Children about Sex and Character*. Westport, CT: Hyperion.

Seecombe, Karen, and Rebecca L. Warner. 2003. *Marriages and Families: Relationships in Social Context*. Fresno, CA: Thomson.

Silverman, Jay G., Anita Raj, Lorelei A. Mucci, and Jeanne E. Hathaway. 2001. "Dating Violence against Adolescent Girls and Associated Substance Use, Unhealthy Weight Control, Sexual Risk Behavior, Pregnancy, and Suicidality." *Journal of the American Medical Association*, 286 (5): 1124–1139.

Simmons, Tavia, and Martin O'Connell. 2003. *Married Couple and Unmarried Partner Households: 2000*. Washington, DC: U.S. Department of Commerce.

Somers, Cheryl L., and Jamie H. Gleason. 2001. "Does Source of Sex Education Predict Adolescents' Sexual Knowledge, Attitudes, and Behaviors?" *Education*, 121 (4): 674–682.

Spirito, Anthony. 2000. "Adolescent Risk-Taking and Self-Reported Injuries Associated with Substance Abuse." *American Journal of Drug and Alcohol Abuse*, 12 (2): 16–25.

Steinberg, Laurence. 2002. *Adolescence (6th Ed.)*. New York: McGraw-Hill.

Stern, Steven E., and Alysia D. Handel. 2001. "Sexuality And Mass

Media: The Historical Context of Psychology's Reaction to Sexuality on the Internet." *Journal of Sex Research*, 38 (4): 22–33.

Stevenson, Michael R., and Jeanine C. Cogan. 2003. *Everyday Activism: A Handbook for Lesbian, Gay, and Bisexual People and Their Allies*. Bristol, PA: Taylor and Francis.

Strasburger, Victor C., and Barbara Wilson. 2002. *Children, Adolescents, and the Media*. Thousand Oaks, CA: Sage.

Terry, Elizabeth, and Jennifer Manlove. 2000. *Trends in Sexual Activity and Contraceptive Use among Teens*. Washington, DC: Child Trends.

Tjaden, Patricia, and Nancy Thoennes. 2000a. *Full Report of the Prevalence, Incidence, and Consequences of Intimate Partner Violence against Women: Findings from the National Violence against Women Survey*. Washington, DC: National Institute of Justice and the Centers for Disease Control and Prevention.

———. 2000b. *Extent, Nature, and Consequences of Intimate Partner Violence: Findings from the National Violence against Women Survey*. Washington, DC: National Institute of Justice and the Centers for Disease Control and Prevention.

U.S. Bureau of the Census. 2003a. Married-Couple and Unmarried-Partner Households. *Census 2000 Special Reports*. Washington, DC: U.S. Government Printing Office.

———. 2003b. *Statistical Abstract of the United States (122nd Ed.)*. Washington, DC: U.S. Government Printing Office.

U.S. Customs Service. 2001. *Ecstasy News: Updated Message to Parents: The Growing Ecstasy Threat*. Retrieved March 29, 2003, from: http://www.customs.ustreas.gov/hot-new/pressrel/ecstasynews.htm.

U.S. Department of Commerce. 2002. *A Nation Online: How Americans Are Expanding Their Use of the Internet*. Washington, DC: Economics and Statistics Administration.

U.S. Department of Justice, Drug Enforcement Administration. 2001. *Drug Intelligence Brief: Club Drugs: An Update*. Retrieved March 29, 2003, from: http://www.dea.gov/pubs/intel/01026/index.html.

U.S. Department of Labor. 2002a. *A Profile of the Working Poor, 2000*. Washington, DC: U.S. Bureau of Labor Statistics.

———. 2002b. *Occupational Outlook Handbook, 2002–2003*. Washington, DC: U.S. Bureau of Labor Statistics.

U.S. Federal Bureau of Investigation. 2002. *Uniform Crime Reports*. Washington, DC: U.S. Department of Justice.

U.S. Food and Drug Administration. 2000. *The Death of the Party: All the Rave, GHB's Hazards Go Unheeded.* Retrieved March 29, 2003, from: http://www.fda.gov/fdac/features/2000/200_ghb.html.

UNAIDS. 2003. *UNAIDS Statement: Forty-Seventh Session of the Commission on the Status of Women.* New York: Author.

UNAIDS/WHO (World Health Organization). 2002. *AIDS Epidemic Update.* Geneva, Switzerland: Author.

United Nations Children's Fund. 2002. *Young People and HIV/AIDS: Opportunity in Crisis.* New York: Author.

Villani, Susan. 2001. "Impact of Media on Children and Adolescents: A 10-Year Review of the Research." *Journal of the American Academy of Child and Adolescent Psychiatry,* 10 (4): 27–41.

Wechsler, Henry, Debra Fulghum, and Bernice Wuethrich. 2002. *Dying to Drink: Confronting Binge Drinking on College Campuses.* Gordonsville, VA: Rodale.

Wilson, Karen, and Jonathan Klein. 2002. "Opportunities for Appropriate Care: Health Care and Contraceptive Use among Adolescents Reporting Unwanted Sexual Intercourse." *Archives of Pediatrics and Adolescent Medicine,* 156 (4): 341–344.

Wolak, Janis, Kimberly Mitchell, and David Finkelhor. 2003. "Escaping or Connecting? Characteristics of Youth Who Form Close Online Relationships." *Journal of Adolescence,* 26 (1): 105–119.

Yancey, Nancy. 2002. *STDs: What You Don't Know Can Hurt You.* Brookfield, CT: Millbrook.

Young, Kimberly S. 2001. *Tangled in the Web: Understanding Cybersex from Fantasy to Addiction.* St. Louis, MO: First Books.

3

Worldwide Perspective

The first two chapters have shown that teenage dating and sexual behavior in the United States today are quite different and distinct from that of past historical eras. Coming of age presents adolescents with an assortment of dizzying expectations and challenges, from learning Internet do's and don'ts to being mindful of safer sex responsibilities and practices. One must realize, too, that the pace of change varies among and within regions of the world. To develop an insightful and richly textured examination of dating and sexual behavior as it exists today, it is important to expand one's knowledge base of multicultural practices and behaviors.

With this in mind, the purpose of this chapter is to explore the international diversity that exists in adolescents' dating and sexual behaviors. The chapter will journey both near and far in an effort to gather information, in the process charting variations in values, traditions, and transitions. It will study the dating behaviors of adolescents from prosperous nations and discover how their behaviors compare to those of teens from impoverished lands. It will "visit" overpopulated as well as underpopulated nations and will spend time "exploring" both Western and Eastern cultures.

Achieving a world perspective is important for several reasons. First, it encourages a sensitive and tolerant outlook on international customs and a closer analysis and appreciation of cultural variations. Also, it discourages the judging of the behaviors and lifestyles of others as inferior or strange. Additionally, a world perspective may reveal information that stimulates and broadens one's own thinking on important topics, such as in international programs in sexuality education or teenage pregnancy prevention.

Finally, a world perspective may provide culturally appropriate ideas to those who work with adolescents from different parts of the world.

The representative nations in this chapter will be presented alphabetically, beginning with Australia and ending with the United Kingdom. Within each discussion, an effort will be made to address where that nation stands with the topics and issues covered in chapter 2, such as patterns of dating and courtship, teenage marriage trends, presence or absence of sexuality education, contraceptive use, and rates of sexually transmitted diseases. It is important to recognize that this is a selective list of countries and that any such discussions are prone to oversimplification. Nonetheless, this is at least a starting point for developing a world perspective on dating and sexual behavior that will show how American customs and conventions compare and contrast with those of teenagers from other lands. The conclusion of the chapter will sum up the findings and identify some common themes and practices.

Australia

Australia is the only continent in the world that is also a country. Australia is a member of the British Commonwealth of Nations and is composed of six states and two mainland territories. The states are New South Wales, Queensland, South Australia, Tasmania, Victoria, and Western Australia. The two mainland territories are the Northern Territory and the Australian Capital Territory. According to recent census figures, Australia has a population of about 19,700,000. A significant majority of the population lives in urban areas (Population Reference Bureau, 2002a).

Most of Australia's population today is of British origin. As far as ethnic groupings are concerned, about 95 percent of the population is European, 4 percent is Asian, and about one percent is aboriginal. The aborigines were the original settlers of Australia, having arrived on the continent about 12,000 years ago from southeast Asia. Almost all Australians are Christians, with the Church of England (Anglican church) being the largest religious group, followed by the Roman Catholic, Methodist, and Presbyterian churches.

The dating and sexual relationships of Australian adolescents tend to follow many of the patterns exhibited by United States teenagers. For example, dating typically begins by early or mid-adolescence and a substantial proportion of Australians are sexually active as teenagers. Growing numbers of Australian teens are influenced by the frequent portrayals of dating and sex in the mass media, which includes television, magazines, movies, music, and the Internet. As in other developed nations, the mass media provide adolescents with an increasingly accessible way to learn and see about sexual behavior, in turn shaping their sexual beliefs and patterns of behavior (Hughes and Stone, 2003; Collins, 1993).

Adolescent males are more sexually active than adolescent females, and the percentages of adolescents who engage in premarital intercourse increases with age. Australian teenagers tend to favor the permissiveness with affection moral standard: they see premarital sex as acceptable, but only with a partner to whom they are emotionally attached. By age 20, about 60 percent of Australian men and 50 percent of women have experienced coitus. Increased sexual activity among the young, and the threat of HIV/AIDS, has prompted many Australian school systems to rethink sexuality education program strategies, resulting in new emphasis being placed on prevention. However, the country's vast land area means that people outside the main metropolitan areas are often extremely isolated from access to any health services, including sexuality education, safer sex practices, and family planning (International Planned Parenthood Federation, 1998).

Similar to adolescents from other nations, many Australian teenagers do not consistently use reliable forms of contraception as they first become sexually active. Though contraception use improves with age, many Australian teens do not initially use birth control for a variety of reasons: lack of knowledge, peer group pressures, failure to plan ahead, and inaccessibility to family planning services. As far as specific types of contraception are concerned, the pill, female sterilization, and condoms are the most popular. In recent years, there has been an increase in latex condom usage, reflecting, at least in part, a safer sex practice aimed at preventing sexually transmitted diseases (Population Reference Bureau, 2002b). Approximately 12,000 Australians are living with HIV/AIDS; approximately 800 of this total were women (Population Reference Bureau, 2002c; United Nations Statistics Division, 2000).

Marriage is not widespread among Australian teenagers, with only 2 percent choosing this lifestyle (United Nations Statistics Division, 2000). The fertility rate among all Australian married couples is also low, with the total number of lifetime births per woman about 1.7 (Population Reference Bureau, 2000a). Australia's fertility rate is below the level of replacement—about 2.1 lifetime births per woman—needed to keep a nation's births and deaths in balance.

In recent years, there has been an increase in cohabitation, particularly among younger couples. Cohabitation is popular among those wishing to establish financial independence, complete an education, or test the feasibility or potential durability of a relationship. Much like cohabitants in the United States, many Australian couples regard this lifestyle as a precursor to marriage, not an alternative. The mean age of Australian women at first marriage is about 26 years; for men, it is 28 years (Population Reference Bureau, 2002a; Costello and Taylor, 1991).

China

China is the third largest country in the world. Only the Russian Federation and Canada are larger in area. China also has the distinction of being the world's most populous country, containing approximately one-quarter of the world's people. China is an ancient civilization and predominantly a rural, low-income country. Despite recent advances in industrialization, much of the country is still relatively undeveloped. Most of the people live in the eastern third of the country, many in the great river valleys and coastal plains.

Though China contains more than fifty ethnic groups, most of the population is Han Chinese, commonly referred to as "Chinese." About five percent of the population is non-Han Chinese, the Zhuang and the Yi being two of the largest minority groups. The Beijing dialect, or Mandarin, is the national language of China. As far as religion is concerned, most Chinese follow a combination of the teachings of Buddhism, Confucianism, and Taoism. Among China's minority religious groups, Islam is widespread, particularly in western regions of the country.

As one might imagine, China is an overpopulated nation. In an effort to curb its population, which in 2002 was estimated to be at almost 1.3 billion, China implemented a one-child policy in 1979: couples pledging to have only one child received a number of government benefits, including monetary bonuses and preferential treatment for housing, health care, education, and job opportunities. The one-child policy is considered controversial, and its implementation has provoked strong resistance over the years. Most critics question the government's right to intervene in a couple's reproductive decision making. However, there is no mistaking the fact that the policy has created a decline in China's fertility rates: Chinese women had an average of 5.8 children in 1970, but this figure had dropped to about 1.8 in 2002. However, given the country's huge number of people, it will take some time for a significant population decline to be realized. It is projected that if fertility rates continue to decline, China can expect to see its 1.3 billion population begin to decline by 2025 (Population Reference Bureau, 2002a; Poston and Yaukey, 1992).

The dating and sexual behaviors of Chinese couples show interesting variations from those practiced in other nations. Prior to the Communist revolution, parents arranged for all dating partners and marriages. Today, only about 10 percent of marriages are prearranged. China's patriarchal society makes dating a traditional affair, including a conservative sexual morality. Premarital sex and cohabitation are frowned upon, as are public displays of affection such as holding hands or kissing. But although premarital sex is discouraged, rates of sexual activity before marriage have increased in recent years, as has sexual activity not involving intercourse (Caron, 1998).

China's demographic planning has implications for the course of intimate relationships. For example, early marriages have always been encouraged in China, the legal age being 16 for women and 18 for men (the founding of the People's Republic brought legislation in 1950 that raised the age to 18 for women and 20 for men). Citing a link between later marriages and lower fertility rates, the government in 1980 set the minimum age at marriage at 20 for women and 22 for men. In 2002, the mean age at marriage for women was 22; it was 24 for men (Population Reference Bureau, 2002b; United Nations Statistics Division, 2000).

Widespread access to contraception is a vital part of China's population planning program. Contraceptive use among women of reproductive age is currently about 85 percent, a significant increase from earlier years (Population Reference Bureau, 2002a). Most Chinese couples use one of three birth control methods: the intrauterine device (IUD), female sterilization, or male sterilization. Many Chinese women also use abortion as a birth control method. Approximately 10 million abortions are performed in China each year. Abortion is provided free of charge there, and

China is the only developing country where mifepristone (a pill used to chemically induce an abortion; known in the United States as RU 486) has been widely introduced into the health care system for the medical termination of pregnancy (United Nations Statistics Division, 2000; International Planned Parenthood Federation, 1998).

Until recently, formal sexuality education programs were nonexistent for China's younger generations. However recent upswings in the spread of HIV/AIDS and other sexually transmitted diseases have resulted in government intervention. For example, World AIDS Day is recognized in China, and the government has implemented an informational campaign to limit the spread of the disease. Although China only recorded its first AIDS case in 1985, in 2002 the number of HIV-infected persons climbed to more than one million. Experts predict that unless effective intervention takes hold, as many 10 million Chinese people will have acquired HIV by the end of this decade (UNAIDS/WHO, 2002; Population Reference Bureau, 2002c).

The success of sexuality education and family planning programs has been handicapped by the traditional Chinese preference for sons and large families. Also, as China's population is distributed across a vast area, it is difficult to make formal education and services accessible to those living in remote, mountainous, and poverty-stricken areas (International Planned Parenthood Federation, 1998).

France

France is the largest country in western Europe and one of the world's most important industrial and agricultural nations. The intellectual and cultural life of France has also impacted other countries for centuries. France has a population of about 59 million people, which is fairly evenly distributed throughout the country. The majority of the population is of the Roman Catholic faith, and French is the primary language. In some border regions, Breton, Basque, Flemish, and German are spoken.

Similar to trends in other developed nations, French teenagers begin dating at early ages. However, although the French may couple early, they wait longer to go to the altar: recent studies show that the mean age of women at first marriage is about 26 years, and for men it is 28 years (Population Reference

Bureau, 2002a). The traditional, patriarchal scope of French married and family life extends to dating and courtship behaviors. For example, men usually take the initiative to ask women out, provide whatever transportation is needed, and absorb the dating costs, at least during the early stages of a relationship. As in other developed nations, sexual content in the media influences adolescent attitudes and behavior. Sexuality is a common media theme, exposing French adolescents to a variety of images related to dating, gender roles, and sexual intimacy.

Sexual experimentation is not uncommon among French teenagers, and most have experienced premarital intercourse by the end of adolescence. The sexual value system of permissiveness with affection is popular among French adolescents. Although birth control among teens has increased in recent years, early contraceptive use tends to be inconsistent. Of the contraceptives available, the Pill and the IUD are popular choices. In recent years, an increase in latex condom usage has also been reported. The latter is most likely due to national efforts to educate teenagers and the general public on the prevention of HIV/AIDS and other sexually transmitted diseases. In 2002, France reported that approximately 100,000 persons were living with HIV/AIDS, and that 27,000 of this total were women (Population Reference Bureau, 2002c; UNAIDS/WHO, 2002).

Although marriage tends to be delayed, it remains a popular lifestyle. Similar to other European nations (e.g., Germany) cohabitation and singlehood are emerging as alternative and acceptable lifestyle options among the French. As far as patterns of cohabitation are concerned, the young are particularly drawn to this lifestyle, although there has recently been an increase in older French cohabitants. As in other nations, an important reason for the increase in singlehood in France is that more young adults are postponing marriage, usually because of educational or career pursuits.

Marriage among French teenagers is not widespread (approximately 8 percent of all marriages involve adolescents), and only 7 percent of all women give birth by age 20. Today, the average woman in France will give birth to 1.9 children, which is below the 2.1 replacement level. In addition to marrying later, French couples are also having their children later. The average woman has her first child at age 29, compared to age 27 a decade ago (Population Reference Bureau, 2002a, 2002b; Sass and Ashford, 2002).

India

India is the seventh largest country in the world. It occupies a land region about one-third the size of the United States, stretching approximately 2,000 miles from north to south. India has more people than any other country in the world except the People's Republic of China. Despite government policies that foster family planning (in 1951, India became the first country in the world to adopt an official policy to slow population growth), India's population swelled to more than 1 billion in 2002 (Population Reference Bureau, 2002a).

The people of India belong to many different races and religions. Most Indians are either Indo-Aryans, Caucasians who reside mostly in the northern regions of India, or Dravidians, darker-skinned people who live mainly in the south. The vast majority of Indians are Hindus, but India also has one of the world's largest Muslim communities. Other religious groups are Christians, Sikhs, Buddhists, and Jains. Fourteen major languages are spoken in India, and these are further differentiated by hundreds of dialects. Of these many variations, Hindi is the official language of India.

Teenage dating and the path to marriage in India show marked contrasts to those of other nations and are steeped in traditional Indian custom. For example, marriage is viewed more as a relationship between two families than between two persons. As parents arrange most marriages, dating as Americans know it rarely exists. Parents often assess the worth (e.g., financial worth, career potential) of their offspring and look for a partner of equivalent value. However, it should be recognized that growing numbers of young people in India are resisting marriages arranged by their parents. Sexual involvement before marriage is forbidden, and total self-restraint is advocated (Caron, 1998; Singhal and Mrinal, 1991).

Couples exchange marital vows in India at early ages, although this is truer for brides than grooms. To illustrate, almost 40 percent of women in India enter a marital union by age 18, compared to only 3 or 4 percent who marry this young in countries such as Germany or Poland. Childbearing also occurs at early ages in India. About one-half of women in India have their first child by age 18. Females with less than a basic education are more apt to become teenage mothers than those with more schooling. The average woman in India gives birth to 3.2 children, down from 4.2 a decade ago (Sass and Ashford, 2002; Alan Guttmacher Institute, 1998; Kumar, 1991).

In recent years, India has experienced a significant increase in abortions, which are legal. Adolescent females in India are less likely than women over age 20 to use effective contraception. Of the available contraceptive methods, female sterilization, condoms, and the Pill are the most popular. A number of reasons can be cited for ineffective contraceptive use, including lack of information, misconceptions, and fear of side effects (Sass and Ashford, 2002). India is also a patriarchal society, with a strong parental preference for male children. This is a deeply rooted tradition, one that dates back for centuries. Sons are especially preferred in remote areas of the country, where they are expected to help in the fields, add to the family income, and offer parents security in old age (United Nations Statistics Division, 2000). In addition to an overpopulation crisis, India is facing an HIV/AIDS epidemic. As of 2002, an estimated 4 million people were living with HIV/AIDS, the second-highest figure in the world after sub-Saharan Africa (UNAIDS/WHO, 2002).

In addition to HIV/ AIDS, reproductive tract infections and sexually transmitted diseases are also prevalent problems, with approximately 43 million reported cases. There is considerable ignorance about HIV infection, particularly in rural areas, despite the educational efforts of organizations such as the Family Planning Association of India (FPAI). Recent intervention by the FPAI has included efforts to improve the status of women, increase male involvement in sexual and reproductive health issues, and connect AIDS education to industry and the workplace (UNAIDS/WHO, 2002; International Planned Parenthood Federation, 1998).

Indonesia

Indonesia is a country in southeast Asia consisting of more than 13,500 islands. The islands, most of which are small, extend across 3,000 miles of the Indian and Pacific oceans and lie between Asia and Australia. The major islands of Indonesia are Java, Sumatra, Kalimantan, Sulawesi, and Irian Jaya. Indonesia is the world's fifth most populous nation, containing almost 217 million people. Its population is expected to reach more than 300 million by 2050 (Population Reference Bureau, 2002b).

The majority of Indonesia's population are Malays, whose

ancestors originated from southeast Asia. There are many different ethnic and cultural groups in Indonesia, including some Arabs, Chinese, and Papuans. Although Indonesian is the official language, as many as 250 different languages are spoken. About 90 percent of Indonesians are Muslim; Hindus, Christians, and Buddhists comprise most of the rest. As Indonesia is an economically underdeveloped nation with little manufacturing, most Indonesians are farmers. Because of this, most of Indonesia's people live in rural areas, many in small villages.

Indonesia has a high proportion of adolescents: approximately 35 percent of its population is teenagers, and only 5 percent of Indonesians are over age 65. Teenagers begin dating at early ages in Indonesia, and partners are usually selected from one's village community or those nearby. There is a small gap between average age at first intercourse (19.8) and age at marriage (19.9). Almost 20 percent of Indonesian females between the ages of 15 and 19 are married, and more than 30 percent of this total have given birth by age 20. However, it should be mentioned that those residing in urban areas tend to marry later than those from rural settings, and women with higher levels of education tend to have children later (Sass and Ashford, 2002; United Nations Statistics Division, 2000).

Although teenagers in Indonesia are in generally good health, early involvement in sexual activity poses certain health risks, such as exposure to sexually transmitted diseases, unintended pregnancies, and complications from pregnancy and childbirth. High infant, child, and maternal mortality rates tend to accompany teenage pregnancies. Having children as a teenager in Indonesia also puts parents at odds with Indonesia's family planning strategies. Although the number of children born to an Indonesian woman during her lifetime has dropped from 5.6 in the 1960s to 2.6 in 2002, the government feels that this figure is still too high (Sass and Ashford, 2002).

Family planning efforts are aimed at increasing contraceptive knowledge, particularly among the uneducated and those residing in rural areas. Of the available methods, injection, oral contraceptives, and the IUD are used most frequently. Abortion is illegal in Indonesia but is permitted only to save a woman's life (Population Reference Bureau, 2002b; United Nations Population Information Network, 2001b).

Health risks posed by HIV/AIDS and other sexually transmitted diseases also impact teenage sexuality. Approximately

120,000 Indonesians were infected with HIV/AIDS in 2002, approximately 27,000 of this total being females. Of concern in recent years are the increasing numbers of Indonesians, including teenagers, who have become injecting drug users (IDUs). HIV prevalence is high among IDUs, who are estimated to number as many as 196,000 Indonesians. According to 2002 research, the vast majority of IDUs are male, and more than two-thirds of them were sexually active. An estimated 9,000 women had been infected with sexually transmitted diseases by men who injected drugs (UNAIDS/WHO, 2002).

Ireland

Ireland is a small, independent nation in northwestern Europe. Officially called the Republic of Ireland, it occupies the southwestern five-sixths of the island of Ireland, one of the two main British Isles. The northeastern sixth of the island makes up Northern Ireland, which is part of the United Kingdom. Ireland is divided into twenty-six counties and has a population of about 3.8 million. Dublin, the capital of Ireland, and Cork, the second largest city, contain about 25 percent of Ireland's total population.

Most of the Irish people are descendants of settlers from centuries ago, including Celts, Vikings, Normans, and the English. About 95 percent of the population is Roman Catholic, unlike neighboring Northern Ireland, where only one-third of the population is Catholic. Most of the remainder in Ireland are Anglican or members of other Protestant religions. English is the predominant language, although some residents speak Gaelic, or Irish. About one-half of the population resides in cities and towns, and the rest live on farms and rural villages. In recent years, Ireland has experienced a drift of the population toward its cities.

Tradition and custom characterize Irish dating relationships, and the influence of the church is apparent in many areas. Younger generations are taught to view life moralistically and to follow the rules of the church without question. The teachings of the church have a particularly strong bearing on adolescent morality and socialization, particularly the molding of attitudes, values, and standards of behavior expected within the community and within intimate relationships.

Dating typically begins during early adolescence, at which time dating activities are generally encouraged and sanctioned by the community. Teenage dating dynamics reflect the patriarchal structure of Irish marriage and family life and embrace traditional gender role activities. Although premarital sexual relations are frowned upon, young men and women are often under peer-group pressure to do otherwise. As in other nations, sex before marriage is more common for adolescent males than females. Rates of teenage pregnancy and sexually transmitted diseases are relatively low in Ireland. In 2000, government officials in Ireland reported about 2,400 cases of HIV/AIDS, 660 of this total being women (United Nations Statistics Division, 2000; Population Reference Bureau, 2000).

As far as family planning is concerned, the average woman gives birth to about 1.9 children over the course of her lifespan. This is slightly below the replacement fertility level necessary to keep births and deaths in balance and to thus maintain population stability. To help ensure a replacement fertility level, the Irish government has implemented a pronatalist policy that includes child tax allowances, maternity grants, and maternity leave packages. Out-of-wedlock births are rare in Ireland, and abortion is only permitted to save a woman's life (Population Reference Bureau, 2002a, 2002b).

Teenage marriages are extremely rare in Ireland, amounting to only 1–2 percent of all marriages. In fact, Irish couples avoid marrying at young ages: the average age at first marriage for women is about 27 years, and for men, 28 years. Although the pursuit of educational and career goals are important reasons for the delay in first marriages, the living arrangements of young people prior to marriage are also influential factors. Ireland tends to have a high percentage of men and women between the ages of 20 and 24 who choose to live with their parents. Although many young adults in other European nations choose more independent living arrangements, their Irish counterparts are less likely to leave home at this time (Population Reference Bureau, 2002a; 2000).

A number of factors help explain such living arrangements. Financial considerations are particularly important: farmland and jobs are often scarce, and few young people can afford to marry and raise children. In some instances, living with one's parents is a way of maintaining the family estate. The limited availability of affordable rental housing looms as another influential factor. Also, some researchers maintain that compared to people in other European nations, the Irish place less of an emphasis on individualism, which might impact the desire for more independent living arrangements. In a related statistic, cohabitation is not widespread in Ireland. Compared to nations such as Sweden and Denmark, where cohabitation represents an extremely popular lifestyle, only a handful of Irish couples choose to live together (Population Reference Bureau, 2002a; McFalls, 1998; Van de Kaa, 1987).

Japan

Japan is a country of more than 3,000 mountainous islands in the Pacific Ocean, extending 2,000 miles from northeast to southwest. Japan lies along the northeastern coast of Asia and faces Russia, Korea, and China. Four major islands comprise most of Japan's territory: Honshu, Hokkaido, Kyushu, and Shikoku. Overall, Japan is a heavily populated country: about 127.4 million persons live crowded in a land area about one-fourth the size of the United States. Despite limited natural resources, Japan is one of the world's most important industrial nations (Population Reference Bureau, 2002a).

The Japanese are a Mongoloid people with a mixture of Malay and Caucasoid stocks. The largest minority group in Japan is Koreans, although there are also groups of Chinese and Europeans. The religion of Japan is Shinto, but four other religions have influenced the course of Japanese life: Buddhism, Confucianism, Taoism, and Christianity.

Adolescent dating and courtship in Japan reflect some interesting trends. At one time, parents arranged most marriages in Japan. Today, however, only about 25 percent of marriages are structured this way. Instead, teenagers are free to select dating partners from the available pool of eligibles, such as at school, in the neighborhood, or at places of employment. Although parents' influence is still important on the dating partners selected, other factors become evident at the couple level: partners' shared interests, physical attraction, personal feelings, peer influence, and economic and class level, to name but a few.

Teenage marriages represent only 1–2 percent of all marriages. Many Japanese couples are choosing to delay marriage: in 2002, the average age at first marriage for women was 27, and, for men, 30. Regarding the living arrangements of married couples, many reside with one partner's parents, although since World War II, the proportion of Japanese multigenerational households has markedly declined. In recent years, the number of divorces in Japan has been increasing, but it remains low by international standards (Sass and Ashford, 2002; Population Reference Bureau, 2000; Haupt and Kane, 1998; McFalls, 1998).

Sex education in Japanese schools is limited, and most teenagers are often left without sufficient family planning information and services. The choice of modern contraceptive methods is also very limited: the Pill, the IUD, injectables, and implants have not been approved for use, and the diaphragm is no longer produced in Japan due to lack of demand. As far as HIV/AIDS rates of infection are concerned, Japan reported 12,000 cases in 2002, including 6,600 women (UNAIDS/WHO, 2002; United Nations Statistics Division, 2000; International Planned Parenthood Federation, 1998).

The Japanese fertility level in 2002 was 1.3, down from 3.7 children in 1950. This figure places Japan below the level of replacement. Japan's movement toward small families can be explained by several factors. Prominent among these are the high costs of raising children, the increased employment of young people, later marriages and birth rates, and a high abortion rate. Couples who live in rural areas and who live with or near parents tend to have more children than other couples. Most Japanese couples have their first baby within the first few years of marriage. Teenage mothers give birth to just 1 percent of all Japanese babies, and most of these babies are conceived out of wedlock (Sass and Ashford, 2002; Population Reference Bureau, 2002b; Ogawa and Retherford, 1993).

Latin America and the Caribbean

Latin America and the Caribbean include Mexico and all of the countries south of it, as far as the southern tip of South America. In addition to Mexico and South America, then, Latin America also includes the nations of Guatemala, El Salvador, Honduras, Nicaragua, Costa Rica, Panama, Belize, and the islands of the Caribbean Sea (known collectively as the West Indies). Combined, this region consists of about 7.9 million square miles, approximately the same land area as the United States and Canada combined. According to recent census figures, Latin America and the Caribbean have a population of about 531 million people (Population Reference Bureau, 2002a).

Most Latin Americans are of European ancestry, many of Portuguese and Spanish descent. Other main population groupings are Indians, who are descendants of the original inhabitants, and blacks, whose ancestors were brought as slaves from Africa by the Portuguese centuries ago. Today, many from Latin America and the Caribbean are *mestizos*—mixed European and Indian people. Depending on the country, one will find considerable variation in these population groupings. For example, Costa Rica is predominantly European, Indians make up the largest population group in Ecuador, and blacks comprise a majority of the population in the West Indies. Regarding religion, most of the population in Latin America is Roman Catholic. About 5 percent of the population are Protestants, Jews, or members of other religious groups.

As far as dating relationships are concerned, it must be kept in mind that multicultural differences exist among the countries of Latin America and the Caribbean, and the potential for diversity needs to be kept in mind. However, it is possible to identify some common dating and courtship themes. For example, courtships tend to be of short duration, and a significant number of young couples either marry or live together in a consensual union. Depending on the country studied, 20–40 percent of women enter either living arrangement while still teenagers. However, rates for either of these lifestyles among women with less than a basic education are approximately three times those with at least seven years of schooling (Population Reference Bureau, 2000; Alan Guttmacher Institute, 1998).

Traditional gender role behaviors characterize Latin American and Caribbean dating relationships, particularly the machismo concept. The concept of machismo regards a man as authoritarian and superior, and a woman is viewed as dependent and secondary. Whereas the man is the principal breadwinner, the woman's primary responsibilities are usually raising a family and maintaining the home. In recent years, though, a growing number of Latin American and Caribbean women have entered the labor force, which correlates with a corresponding increase in levels of female education. However, even when the woman works outside the home, she is usually expected to handle the housework and child rearing as well. Thus, although social change has helped to erode certain aspects of machismo, it has not disappeared completely (Sass and Ashford, 2002; United Nations Statistics Division, 2000; Ardia, 1991).

Approximately 60 percent of both married and unmarried people are likely to use contraception, with female sterilization, the Pill, and the condom being the most popular choices. The fertility rate in Latin America and the Caribbean is about 2.7. Approximately 35 percent of women give birth to at least one child by the end of adolescence (Population Reference Bureau, 2002b; Sass and Ashford, 2002).

Early sexual activity increases the risk for contracting a sexually transmitted disease, including HIV/AIDS. As of 2002, approximately 1.9 million adults and children living in Latin America and the Caribbean were living with HIV/AIDS. In Latin American countries, HIV infections are concentrated among gay males, prostitutes, and injecting drug users (IDUs). In the Caribbean, where HIV prevalence rates are among the highest in the world, heterosexual contact has been the primary path for HIV transmission. HIV/AIDS is particularly widespread in Haiti and Bermuda (Population Reference Bureau, 2002c; UNAIDS/WHO, 2002).

The Middle East and North Africa

The Middle East and north Africa are land regions covering parts of southwestern Asia, southeastern Europe, and northern Africa. According to recent estimates, the population of the Middle East and north Africa is about 385 million. The population more than doubled between 1970 and 2002, rising from 173 million people to its current total. The population is growing by 2 percent per year (or nearly 7 million people per year), a rate second only to that of sub-Saharan Africa (Population Reference Bureau, 2002a).

The Middle East and north Africa are an extremely complex and diverse part of the world. Much of the region is desert, and most of the people are poor farmers. Most of the people are Arab, but other population groups include Africans, Armenians, Copts, Greeks, Iranians, Jews, Kurds, and Turks. Most Middle Easterners are Muslims. Christians represent the second largest religious group in the Middle East, including Coptic, Greek Orthodox, and Maronite branches. Most Israelis practice Judaism. Arabic is the major spoken language, although the Israelis speak Hebrew.

Given such vast diversities in the Middle East and north Africa, any efforts to explore dating and sexuality in this area represent a simplification. The Middle East and north Africa, much like other regions of the world, are not homogeneous, nor are its teenagers or the relationships they forge. Nonetheless, one can at least identify some general trends and themes.

Teenagers from the Middle East and north Africa are living in a region having a young age structure. About one-third of the region's population is under age 15, and an unprecedented number of young women are reaching reproductive age. Even if these women have fewer children than their parents did, their sheer numbers mean that there will be a large number of children in the near future, giving momentum to population growth in the region. In Jordan, for example, where 40 percent of the population is under age 15, the population is expected to more than double in the next 50 years, from 4.9 million people in 2000 to 11.7 million people in 2050 (Population Reference Bureau, 2002a, 2002b; Sass and Ashford, 2002).

Teenagers are taught that marriage is customary in the Middle East and north Africa, and sexual abstinence is stressed. Dating relationships as well as marriage and family life reflect a strong patriarchal structure. Intermarriage within families (including among first cousins) is prevalent in the Middle East and north Africa, and some communities practice polygyny (Islamic law, for example, allows men to have up to four wives if they can provide adequate justification and they treat all wives equitably). At one time, many adolescent marriages occurred, but the mean age at first marriage for couples has increased in such nations as Iran (22 for women; 25 for men), Turkey (24; 26), and Israel (24; 28). Increased education, particularly among women, as well as financial restraints are among the forces creating this marriage pattern (United Nations Statistics Division, 2000; Haupt and Kane, 1998; McFalls, 1998).

Adolescents in these nations are also taught that unlike in other nations, cohabitation is an unacceptable living arrangement in Islamic culture and is rare even among non-Muslims in the Middle East. Also, once marriage has taken place, it is not uncommon for the bride and groom to be joined by a number of different relatives to live under the same roof. For example, some couples might share a home with parents or grandparents; others might live with brothers, sisters, uncles, and aunts; and still other homes reflect a combination of the foregoing. As domestic authority is a male province, extended households are headed by the husband, grandfather, or an uncle (Omran and Roudi, 1993).

As far as Middle Eastern and north African fertility rates are concerned, the average woman gives birth to about 3.6 children. However, considerable variation in fertility rate exists among nations in this region. For example, the fertility rate ranges from 2.9 children in Israel to 4.1 in Syria and 5.4 in Iraq. Religion also figures prominently in a woman's fertility rate, as large families are encouraged in Islamic culture (Sass and Ashford, 2002; Population Reference Bureau, 2000b).

Although family planning is permitted under Islamic law, contraceptive use tends to be low in the Middle East and north Africa. Similar to trends in other parts of the world, educated women living in urban areas are more likely than rural women to practice birth control. The Pill, the IUD, and the condom tend to be popular choices. Most Middle Eastern and north African countries do not allow abortion as a family planning measure (United Nations Statistics Division, 2000; Myers and Agree, 1994; Omran, 1992).

Sexually active adolescents face a number of reproductive health issues, including high maternal mortality (particularly in Yemen, Morocco, Egypt, and Iraq) and the increasing prevalence of sexually transmitted diseases, especially HIV/AIDS. Regarding the latter, in 2002 an estimated 550,000 people were living with HIV/AIDS in this region, and 37,000 lives were claimed by the epidemic. Recent significant outbreaks of HIV infections among injecting drug users have occurred in north Africa and Iran (UNAIDS/WHO, 2002; Population Reference Bureau, 2002c).

The Russian Federation

The Russian Federation, formerly known as the Soviet Union, is located in northern Asia, bordering the Arctic Ocean, between Europe and the northern Pacific Ocean. It occupies a land mass of more than 6.5 million square miles, which makes it slightly more than 1.8 times the size of the United States. The Russian Federation is a democratic republic formed in 1991 from the Russian Soviet Federative Socialist Republic of the Soviet Union. The current Russian Federation constitution was adopted in 1993 by national referendum. It has a population of approximately 144 million people (Population Reference Bureau, 2002a).

The people of the Russian Federation are quite diverse and represent more than 100 officially recognized ethnic groups. Only one-half of the people in the Russian Federation are ethnically Russian; that is, speaking Russian as a native language or having family roots in Russia. The other one-half consists of a wide range of population groups, from the European, mostly Christian Estonians, to the central Asian, Islamic Uzbeks. Although Russians have settled in every location of the country, different nationalities form the majority in all of the national republics that now constitute the Russian Federation. The primary religion of the Russian Federation is Orthodox Christian, and Islam is the second largest religious group.

Russian teenagers date for the same reasons given by adolescents in other countries: recreation, friendship, companionship, sexual experimentation, and mate selection. Compared to earlier times, Russian teenagers tend to date earlier and initiate sexual activity earlier. Although sexuality education for teenagers exists, it is not widespread at the present time. Unprotected sexual intercourse is common among adolescents, and rates of sexually transmitted diseases and teen pregnancies have increased in recent years.

Dating in Russia paves the way for the country's high marriage rate, a reflection of the emphasis placed on family life. Unlike the trends of delayed marriage reported in this chapter for some other countries (e.g., Australia, France, and Ireland), Russian couples tend to marry at earlier ages: an average age of 23 for women and 25 for men. Approximately 13 percent of all marriages involve teenagers (Population Reference Bureau, 2002a; Sass and Ashford, 2002).

As far as family planning is concerned, the average Russian woman gives birth to about 1.3 children. This is far below the 2.1 level of replacement needed to stabilize a population, a level last realized by Russia in 1988. Despite the implementation of pronatalist policies such as extended and paid maternity leave and easier qualification for parents in acquiring housing and other benefits, the fertility rate has steadily declined to its present level. Russia's population of 144 million is down 4.3 million from its peak at the beginning of 1992.

Contraceptive use by both unmarried and married Russians is low, and birth control is not always readily available. Because of this, abortion is the leading form of birth control, especially among adolescents. In fact, Russia has the highest abortion rate in the world. On average, Russian women experience 4–5 abortions during their reproductive lifetimes. There is evidence (Creel,

2002), however, that abortion rates may be declining, at least in some neighboring regions. Kazakhstan, Kyrgyzstan and Uzbekistan, which became independent states in 1991, report that rates of induced abortion have decreased in those countries since the dissolution of the Soviet Union. Since this has happened, there has been a corresponding increase in the use of contraceptives such as the IUD. Whether this trend spreads throughout the Russian Federation, however, remains to be seen (Creel, 2002; Population Reference Bureau, 2002b; International Planned Parenthood Federation, 1998; Zhernova, 1991).

Sexually transmitted diseases have sharply increased among Russian teenagers in recent years, most notably syphilis and gonorrhea. An increase in sexual permissiveness, sexual activity at earlier ages, lack of sexuality education emphasizing prevention, and an absence of latex condoms are major contributing factors. The Russian Federation also has one of the sharpest increases of HIV/AIDS in the world. As of 2002, the number of persons living with HIV/AIDS was estimated to be at 700,000, 180,000 of this total being women. This is a profound increase from 1998, when about 11,000 cases were reported. In less than eight years, HIV/AIDS epidemics have been discovered in more than thirty cities and in eighty-six of Russia's eighty-nine regions. Up to 90 percent of new HIV cases have been attributed to use of injected drugs (UNAIDS/WHO, 2002; Population Reference Bureau, 2002c).

Sub-Saharan Africa

Sub-Saharan Africa consists of forty-two nations located south of the Sahara. This land region occupies approximately 20 percent of the Earth's land surface and contains a population estimated in 2002 to be almost 700 million, or approximately 10 percent of the world's population. By 2025, this total is expected to eclipse 1 billion. More than 60 percent of this population lives in Nigeria, Ghana, Sudan, Uganda, Zaire, and Zambia (Population Reference Bureau, 2002a).

Sub-Saharan Africa also has considerable population diversity. There are approximately 800 ethnic groups speaking more than 1,000 different languages or dialects. Although millions of Africans are of mixed origins, the population includes five major physical types: Negroid, Pygmoid, Bushmanoid, Caucasoid, and Mongoloid. Many African religions are tribal religions; however,

Islam is becoming increasingly popular. Sub-Saharan Africa has also experienced an increase in various Christian churches.

The population of sub-Saharan Africa is a young one, with almost 45 percent of its people under age 15 and just 3 percent over age 65. The life expectancy in most countries in sub-Saharan Africa is barely fifty years. The population of sub-Saharan Africa includes approximately 70 million teenagers between the ages of 15 and 19 (Population Reference Bureau, 2002c).

Although a number of factors contribute to Africans' shortened life expectancy (e.g., malnutrition, poor sanitation, and limited health care services), a major cause is the high prevalence rates of HIV/AIDS. A total of almost 30 million people are infected by this disease, making sub-Saharan Africa the hardest-hit region in the world. Because the virus is spread primarily through heterosexual activity, the number of HIV-infected women approximates the number of men, although in 2002 the figure for women increased to 55 percent of all cases. Approximately 3.5 million new infections were diagnosed in 2002, and the epidemic took the lives of an estimated 2.4 million Africans. About 10 million people between the ages of 15 and 24 and almost 3 million children under 15 are living with HIV (UN/AIDS, 2002; Population Reference Bureau, 2002c).

Adolescent courtship tends to occupy a short period of time, and many Africans enter marriage at young ages. To illustrate, the average age at first marriage for women in all of sub-Saharan Africa is 19, and it is as young as 16 in Nigeria and northern regions of Sudan (Sass and Ashford, 2002). Marriage is often seen as a contract between families, with reproductive rights belonging to the husband and his family. Polygyny is not uncommon in some sub-Saharan countries; for example, about 45 percent of married women in Mali and 38 percent in Liberia live in such arrangements. However, polygyny is an expensive venture, and few men have the finances to support several wives and even more children (United Nations Statistics Division, 2000; Okafor, 1991).

As far as family planning is concerned, sub-Saharan Africa has the highest population growth rate of any region on Earth, almost three percent annually. Overall, the fertility rate of a woman in sub-Saharan Africa is 5.6, well above the level of replacement. It should be recognized, though, that fertility rates vary within the various countries of sub-Saharan Africa. For example, the average Rwandan woman will give birth to 5.8 children over the course of her lifetime, but the corresponding figure for women in

Niger is 8.0. The fertility rate is lower in Lesotho and Swaziland, 4.3 and 4.5, respectively. A number of factors account for such large families such as poverty (which is linked to limited access to and knowledge of family planning) and early marriage, to name but a few (Population Reference Bureau, 2002a, 2002b; Sass and Ashford, 2002).

Early sexual activity and poor contraceptive use make adolescents in sub-Saharan Africa a vulnerable group. A majority of the teenage population has had premarital sex before age 20. It is estimated that no more than 20 percent of the teenage population utilizes reliable birth control. Furthermore, research consistently shows (e.g., Population Reference Bureau, 2002b) that young African females are dangerously undereducated about HIV/AIDS and how to protect themselves from it. Even worse, HIV prevalence rates among pregnant women continue to soar upward. For instance, HIV prevalence among pregnant women in urban Botswana rose from 39 percent to 45 percent between 1997 and 2001 (UNAIDS/WHO, 2002; Sass and Ashford, 2002; Population Reference Bureau, 2002c).

Sweden

Sweden, also known as the Kingdom of Sweden, is one of the Scandinavian countries of northern Europe. It occupies the eastern half of the Scandinavian peninsula and is bordered by Norway and Finland. Sweden is the fourth largest country in Europe, a bit larger in size than the state of California. However, Sweden is thinly populated and has one of the world's lowest population growth rates. Its population is about 9 million, most of which is concentrated in urban areas, particularly in southern regions of the nation (Population Reference Bureau, 2002a).

Most of Sweden's people are ethnically and culturally homogenous, although there are small minorities of Lapps and Finns in the north. Swedes are closely related to the Danes and Norwegians. The universal language is Swedish, a Germanic tongue that resembles Danish and Norwegian. The dominant religion is Lutheranism; other religious groups include the Missionary Union, the Pentecostal Movement, Baptists, Roman Catholics, and Jews.

Swedish adolescents grow up in a nation experiencing sweeping lifestyle changes, some so dramatic that many feel that the institutions of marriage and family life have been redefined. As with other nations, dating in Sweden typically begins during early adolescence, but relationship dynamics tend to be more egalitarian than traditional. This means there is a mixing of male and female roles rather than sex-typed expectations. Sweden has very liberal attitudes toward adolescent sexuality, and most teens have lost their virginity by age 17. Many Swedish teenagers believe in the permissiveness with affection sexual standard, in which sexual activity is viewed as acceptable provided the partners are emotionally connected (Population Reference Bureau, 2000; Caron, 1998; Haupt and Kane, 1998).

Swedish teenagers also find that courtship does not always lead to marriage: it is estimated that, in the years to come, only 60 percent of Swedish men and women will ever marry. This means that modern Swedish couples are less likely to marry than couples from any other industrialized nation. Should marriage take place, Swedes are also more likely to delay getting married. The mean age of first marriage is about 31 for women and 33 for men. Teenage marriages are also extremely rare, with teens representing less than 1 percent of the married population. Interestingly, the mean age of Swedish women at first marriage is now higher than the mean age of Swedish women at first birth. Because of this, it not uncommon for children to be present at their parents' first wedding ceremony (Population Reference Bureau, 2002a; Sass and Ashford, 2002; Haupt and Kane, 1998; McFalls, 1998).

Swedish adolescents are also living in a nation experiencing widespread cohabitation, a lifestyle choice that many feel has become a part of the courtship process. Sweden was among the first countries to accept and adopt this lifestyle, uncommon until the end of the 1960s. Unlike in the United States, cohabitation in Sweden is usually not a prelude to marriage. Rather, it has become a lifestyle in and of itself. Instead of being a trial marriage, it is regarded by many Swedish couples as a distinct alternative to marriage. In addition to being a popular alternative lifestyle for adults, cohabitation has also affected Sweden's fertility picture: about one-half of all births in Sweden are to unmarried parents (Haupt and Kane, 1998; Van de Kaa, 1987; Popenoe, 1987).

In addition to low marriage rates and an increase in cohabitation, Sweden also has a high divorce rate (one can only speculate about how many nonmarital cohabitation relationships dissolve). This has resulted in a large number of single parent households, mostly headed by women. Divorced Swedes also demonstrate a general reluctance to remarry. Many divorced or widowed men and women are now opting to remain single rather than entering another marriage. With the widespread acceptance of cohabitation, not marrying or remarrying has become a legitimate lifestyle option. For that matter, more relaxed divorce laws make it easier to obtain a divorce in Sweden and other nations than it was generations ago (Haupt and Kane, 1998; Van de Kaa, 1987).

All of the foregoing Swedish lifestyle trends have resulted in a small family size in the country. Women give birth to an average of 1.6 children, a fertility rate that places Sweden below the level of replacement. Contraceptives are easily accessible and affordable, and they are without religious prohibition. Abortion is legal up to the end of 18 weeks of pregnancy without restriction as to reason, but Sweden has one of the lowest abortion rates in the world. Rates of sexually transmitted diseases, including HIV/AIDS, are also low. Sweden reported 3,300 cases of persons living with HIV/AIDS in 2002, with 880 women being part of this total (UNAIDS/WHO, 2002; Population Reference Bureau, 2002c).

Experts maintain that Sweden's success in the aforementioned areas is a result of its national sexuality education program, which is compulsory in Sweden's schools and begins when a child is eight years old. Employing an age-appropriate curriculum, Sweden supplies children and teenagers with information on a variety of important sexuality topics, including family planning, the prevention of sexually transmitted diseases, sexual and reproductive health rights, and the enjoyment of sexual expression (Population Reference Bureau, 2000; International Planned Parenthood Federation, 1998; Caron, 1998).

United Kingdom

The United Kingdom, known officially as the United Kingdom of Great Britain and Northern Ireland, is a union of four countries: England, Scotland, Wales, and Northern Ireland. Commonly referred to as Great Britain or Britain, the United Kingdom encompasses most of the British Isles, which are located off the northwest coast of continental Europe. The combined population of the United Kingdom is about 61 million (Population Reference Bureau, 2002a).

Most Britons are descendants of Celtic, French, Germanic, and Scandinavian peoples. Among the few minority groups are people from the West Indies and Asia. English is the universal language, although Welsh and Gaelic are spoken in some northern regions. The United Kingdom has two national churches: the Church of England, which is Episcopal, and the Church of Scotland, which is Presbyterian. Other important religions are Roman Catholicism and various Protestant denominations, such as Baptist and Methodist.

Similar to other developed nations, dating in the United Kingdom begins at early ages, and teens are under strong social and peer group pressure to engage in premarital sex. Many Britons favor the permissiveness with affection sexual standard. Many features of modern life in the United Kingdom increase both the desire and the opportunity for adolescent sexual activity: the mass media; the breakdown of traditional values such as abstinence; and the increase of permissiveness, urbanization, and materialism. Although increasing numbers of couples practice egalitarianism in the United Kingdom, adolescent dating dynamics tend to capture a traditional and conventional style as well as the patriarchal structure characterizing marriage and family life. Sexuality education in the United Kingdom is a part of the curriculum through secondary school (Population Reference Bureau, 2000; Alan Guttmacher Institute, 1998).

Marriage is considered important in the United Kingdom, a fact evidenced by one of the highest marriage rates in northern Europe. Dating and courtship are marked by freedom of choice, and most Britons choose partners who are within relatively close residential proximity. Should marriage be in the picture, Britons are similar to their northern European neighbors and delay the exchange of wedding vows until about 26 years of age for women and 28 years for men. Adolescent marriages represent only 3 percent of all marriages. Although rates of cohabitation and singlehood have increased, most notably in England, they have not nearly reached the levels of popularity demonstrated in such countries as Sweden or Denmark (Population Reference Bureau, 2002a; Sass and Ashford, 2002; United Nations Population Information Network, 2001a; Lowenstein and Lowenstein, 1991).

Since the 1970s, Britons have been having fewer children. Currently, the average woman in the United Kingdom gives birth to 1.7 children over the course of her reproductive years. This is another example of a developed nation falling below the level of replacement and not maintaining the number of births needed to keep births and deaths in balance (and thus ensure population stability). A number of reasons can be cited for the United Kingdom's fertility decline, including financial considerations, more efficient contraceptives, relaxation of abortion laws in the late 1960s, and educational and vocational commitments (Population Reference Bureau, 2002b; Haupt and Kane, 1998; McFalls, 1998; Van de Kaa, 1987).

As far as family planning methods in the United Kingdom are concerned, women traditionally assume the responsibility for birth control. Oral contraceptives are a popular form of birth control, followed by condoms. In recent years, there has been an increase in both female and male sterilization, particularly among married couples. Abortion is legal in the United Kingdom up to 24 weeks into the pregnancy. The United Kingdom offers a variety of family planning information to teenagers as well as to the general public. For example, the United Kingdom Family Planning Association (UKFPA) focuses on information related to birth control and fertility awareness, as well as education on sexually transmitted diseases (Sass and Ashford, 2002; United Nations Population Information Network, 2001b; International Planned Parenthood Federation, 1998).

In recent years, there has been an increase in the rates of sexually transmitted diseases, including HIV/AIDS. As of 2002, the number of persons living with HIV/AIDS was 34,300, with 7,400 of this total being women. Several new trends regarding the disease have recently become evident. For one, more than one-half of the 4,279 new HIV infections in 2001 resulted from heterosexual sex, compared to 33 percent of new infections in 1998. In addition, a large share of these infections were diagnosed in persons who originated from, or who have lived in or visited, areas where HIV prevalence is high. Given these scenarios, the United Kingdom recognizes that prevention, treatment, and care activities of persons with HIV/AIDS need to become more culturally appropriate and socially relevant if they are to reach and benefit such diverse communities (UNAIDS/WHO, 2002; Population Reference Bureau, 2002c).

Summary

After completing this abbreviated journey around the globe, this section of the chapter will briefly summarize the findings. One of the more obvious facts is that from a global perspective, dating represents the primary social vehicle for pair bonding, a conscious and deliberate process of mate selection. In developed as well as developing nations, dating typically begins during adolescence and is often prompted by encouragement of early heterosexual interactions in neighborhoods, schools, or at social functions.

In developed nations, including the United States, media images of dating and sexual behaviors shape the values, beliefs, and behaviors of young generations. Although urbanized, developed nations bring many advantages to teenagers, such as heightened educational opportunities and access to health services, modernization also has the potential of exposing adolescents to such negative influences as illicit drugs and sexually transmitted diseases.

A global investigation uncovers some fairly universal dating and sexual behaviors. For example, just as in the United States, a patriarchal structure tends to characterize most relationships in other countries. Although teens from some nations (e.g., France, Sweden) practice some degree of egalitarianism, courtship in most countries reflects traditional gender roles. The permissiveness with affection sexual value orientation is widespread around the globe. Cohabitation is especially popular in developed regions of the world, such as France and Sweden, but it is met with resistance in parts of China, the Middle East, and north Africa. Along similar lines, although delayed marriages are common in developed parts of the world, earlier marriages tend to characterize developing nations. Finally, teenage marriages are not widespread in developed nations, but they are commonplace in regions such as sub-Saharan Africa, where family planning is scarce and a shortened life cycle prevails.

In virtually all of the nations "visited" in this chapter, an ever-increasing percentage of adolescents are engaging in sexual activity, and they are doing so at earlier ages. For the most part, teenagers do not consistently use reliable forms of contraception, although this is truer for younger teens and for those with limited education than it is for their older, better-educated counterparts. It is also apparent from the discussions in this chapter how involvement in sexual activity brings the potential for various health risks, such as unintended pregnancy, complications from abortion or childbirth, and infection from sexually transmitted diseases.

No teenager in any country is immune from the ravages of HIV/AIDS, although this disease has struck hardest in sub-Saharan Africa, China, eastern Europe, Asia, and the Pacific. As this epidemic continues to spread, people of all ages need access to services and information to protect them against HIV/AIDS. Among the world's adolescents, this underscores the need for comprehensive and accurate information about STD prevention, as well as about other important sexuality topics, including contraception, family planning, pregnancy, communication skills, and values clarification.

References

Alan Guttmacher Institute. 1998. *Into a New World: Young Women's Sexual and Reproductive Lives.* New York: Author.

Ardia, Ruben. 1991. "Women in Latin America." In Leonore L. Adler (Ed.), *Women in Cross-Cultural Perspective.* Westport, CT: Praeger.

Caron, Sandra L. 1998. *Cross-Cultural Perspectives on Human Sexuality.* Needham Heights, MA: Allyn and Bacon.

Coale, Ansley J., Wang Feng, Nancy E. Riley, and Lin Fu De. 1991. "Recent Trends in Fertility and Nuptiality in China." *Science,* 251, 389–393.

Collins, John K. 1993. "Approaches to Adolescent Sexuality: The Australian Picture." *Australian Journal of Marriage and Family,* 14, 14-32.

Costello, Brian R., and Janet Lee Taylor. 1991. "Women in Australia." In Leonore L. Adler (Ed.), *Women in Cross-Cultural Perspective.* Westport, CT: Praeger.

Creel, Liz. 2002. "A Fading Abortion Culture in Three Central Asian Republics." *Demographic and Health Surveys Program,* 10 (April), 11–17.

Haupt, Arthur, and Thomas Kane. 1998. *Population Handbook: International Edition (4th Ed.).* Washington, DC: Population Reference Bureau.

Hughes, Jody and Wendy Stone. 2003. "Family Change and Community Life: Exploring the Links." *Australian Institute of Family Studies,* 4, 1-41.

International Planned Parenthood Federation. 1998. *Country Profiles.* London: Author.

Kumar, Usha. 1991. "Life Stages in the Development of the Hindu Woman in India." In Leonore L. Adler (Ed.), *Women in Cross-Cultural Perspective.* Westport, CT: Praeger.

Lowenstein, Ludwig F., and Kathleen Lowenstein. 1991. "Women in Great Britain." In Leonore L. Adler (Ed.), *Women in Cross-Cultural Perspective.* Westport, CT: Praeger.

McFalls, Joseph. 1998. *Population: A Lively Introduction (3rd Ed.)*. Washington, DC: Population Reference Bureau.

Myers, George C., and Emily M. Agree. 1994. "The World Ages, the Family Changes: A Demographic Perspective." *Ageing International*, 21, 11–18.

Ogawa, Naohiro, and Robert D. Retherford. 1993. "The Resumption of Fertility Decline in Japan." *Population and Development Review*, 19, 703–741.

Okafor, Nmutaka A. O. 1991. "Some Traditional Aspects of Nigerian Women." In Leonore L. Adler (Ed.), *Women in Cross-Cultural Perspective*. Westport, CT: Praeger.

Omran, Abdel R. 1992. *Family Planning in the Legacy of Islam*. New York: Routeledge.

Omran, Abdel R., and Farzaneh Roudi. 1993. *The Middle East Population Puzzle*. Washington, DC: Population Reference Bureau.

Popenoe, David. 1987. "Beyond the Nuclear Family: A Statistical Portrait of the Changing Family in Sweden." *Journal of Marriage and the Family*, 49, 173–183.

Population Reference Bureau. 2000. *The World's Youth 2000*. Washington, DC: Author.

Population Reference Bureau. 2002a. *2002 World Population Data Sheet*. Washington, DC: Author.

Population Reference Bureau. 2002b. *Family Planning Worldwide*. Washington, DC: Author.

Population Reference Bureau. 2002c. *Facing the HIV/AIDS Pandemic*. Washington, DC: Author.

Poston, Dudley L., and David Yaukey. 1992. *The Demography of Modern China*. New York: Plenum.

Sass, Justine, and Lori Ashford. 2002. *2002 Women of Our World*. Washington, DC: Population Reference Bureau.

Singhal, Uma, and Nihar R. Mrinal. 1991. "Tribal Women on India: The Tharu Women." In Leonore L. Adler (Ed.), *Women in Cross-Cultural Perspective*. Westport, CT: Praeger.

UNAIDS /WHO (World Health Organization). 2002. *AIDS Epidemic Update*. Geneva, Switzerland: Author.

United Nations Population Information Network. 2001a. *World Population Prospects*. New York: Author.

United Nations Population Information Network. 2001b. *World Contraceptive Use*. New York: Author.

United Nations Statistics Division. 2000. *The World's Women 2000: Trends and Statistics.* New York: Author.

Van de Kaa, Dirk. 1987. *Europe's Second Demographic Transition.* Washington, DC: Population Reference Bureau.

Zhernova, Lena. 1991. "Women in the USSR." In Leonore L. Adler (Ed.), *Women in Cross-Cultural Perspective.* Westport, CT: Praeger.

4

Chronology

This chapter provides a historical chronology of innovations, milestones, and government legislation shaping adolescent dating and sexuality, from the beginning of the twentieth century to the present day. Any effort to create such a timeline is, of course, selective and prone to oversimplification. But, this timeline captures the diversity of events impacting the teenage experience in the United States, such as research contributions, mass media developments, inventions, recreational pursuits, birth control innovations, and trends in sexually transmitted diseases. As such, this timeline will complement and extend the material contained in other chapters of the book.

1900   The intrauterine device (IUD), a female contraceptive, is invented in Germany.

Sigmund Freud publishes *Interpretation of Dreams.*

1905   The first movie theater opens in Pittsburgh.

1906   The jukebox is invented in Chicago and can play up to twenty-four songs.

1908   Assembly line production of Henry Ford's Model T automobile begins; over the next 20 years, 18 million of these cars will be mass-produced.

1911   Pennsylvania becomes the first state to institute film censorship laws.

1916   The first birth control clinic, founded by Margaret Sanger, opens in Brooklyn, New York.

1917   The United States enters World War I; the "War to End All Wars" ends in 1918.

1920   Ratification of the nineteenth Amendment gives women the right to vote.

         Prohibition goes into effect in the United States, making it illegal to manufacture, transport, or sell alcoholic beverages. Prohibition will be repealed in 1933.

         Singer Bessie Smith helps to popularize blues music.

         The first experimental Technicolor film is developed.

1921   Margaret Sanger and Mary Ware Dennett found the American Birth Control League, which will eventually become the Planned Parenthood Federation of America.

         D. H. Lawrence's *Women in Love* examines the complexities of intimate relationships.

         The first Miss America Pageant is held in Atlantic City, New Jersey.

1922   Emily Post publishes *Etiquette in Society, in Business, in Politics and at Home.*

         Louis Armstrong and Duke Ellington help to popularize jazz music.

1924   At this point, 3 million radios exist in the United States.

1925   Country and western music is popularized at the Grand Ole Opry in Nashville, Tennessee.

1926   Hugh Heffner (eventual publisher of *Playboy* magazine) is born in Chicago.

1928   The Charleston becomes the new dance craze.

D. H. Lawrence's *Lady Chatterly's Lover* is banned for its "graphic" sexual content.

The first scheduled television broadcasts are aired.

1929   The stock market crash occurs; the Great Depression begins and will last ten years.

Bertrand Russell publishes *Marriage and Morals*.

First FM radio broadcasts are made.

The first Academy Awards are announced.

The majority of American families own an automobile.

1930   The "Golden Age" of radio begins.

The pinball machine is marketed in the United States.

The Motion Picture Producers and Distributors of America establish a "code of decency" for what is considered acceptable in films.

1932   The marriage rate is down by 22 percent; the birth rate is down by 15 percent.

1933   One-quarter of American workers are unemployed.

The first drive-in theater opens in Camden, New Jersey.

British researcher Henry Havelock Ellis publishes *Studies in the Psychology of Sex*.

1935   Anthropologist Margaret Mead publishes *Sex and Temperament in Three Primitive Societies*, in which she explores the many sides to gender relations.

Clarinetist Benny Goodman is named music's "King of Swing."

1936   The electric guitar is invented.

1937   The American Medical Association officially recognizes birth control as an integral part of medical practice and education.

1938   Strobe lighting is invented.

           Currently, 50 million radios operate in the United States.

1940   Big bands headline popular music.

1941   The United States enters World War II, which will last until 1945.

           Television broadcasting begins in the United States.

1943   More than 300,000 women are employed by the U.S. aircraft industry.

           Wartime propaganda urges women to join the labor force for the duration of World War II.

           The Jitterbug becomes a new dance craze.

1945   More than 6,000,000 American women are in the labor force by the middle of World War II.

1946   The nation's baby boom is in full swing; more marriages take place than in any other year.

           The United States has 1,000 licensed radio stations.

1947   The Institute for Sex Research, later to be renamed the Kinsey Institute, is established at Indiana University.

1948   Alfred Kinsey publishes *Sexual Behavior of the Human Male*.

           Americans buy 100,000 television sets per week.

1949   The 45-rpm record and record player is manufactured by RCA.

1950   The United States enters the Korean War, which will last until 1953.

        The average home in the United States has two radios.

1951   The Motion Pictures Production Code specifically prohibits films dealing with abortion or narcotics.

        Novelist J. D. Salinger writes the controversial *Catcher in the Rye.*

1952   The transistor radio is invented.

        American Bandstand debuts on television.

1953   *Playboy* magazine debuts.

        Alfred Kinsey publishes *Sexual Behavior of the Human Female.*

1954   Approximately 54 percent of American homes have a television set.

        TV Guide debuts.

        Elvis Presley becomes the United States' first rock and roll star.

        Color television broadcasts begin.

1955   *Blackboard Jungle* is the first film to feature a rock and roll song, Bill Haley's *Rock around the Clock.*

        Teenage idol James Dean dies in a car crash at age 26.

        Chuck Berry records the hit *Maybellene.*

1956   Elvis Presley stars in his first film, *Love Me Tender.*

        Novelist Grace Metalious publishes the steamy novel *Peyton Place.*

1956,   The ABC Radio Network bans Billie Holiday's rendition
cont.   of Cole Porter's *Love for Sale* from all of its stations be-
        cause of its prostitution theme. Stations continue to play
        instrumental versions of the song.

1957   The word "beatnik" is used to describe the emerging
        "Beat Generation" counterculture movement.

        Producers of the *Ed Sullivan Show* instruct camera opera-
        tors to show Elvis Presley only from the waist up on his
        third and final appearance on the program.

1958   Stereo records are manufactured in the United States.

1959   The microchip is invented.

        The first Grammy Awards are recognized by the record-
        ing industry.

        Rock stars Buddy Holly, Ritchie Valens, and J. P. "Big
        Bopper" Richardson die in an Iowa plane crash.

        The Motown record company is created.

        The Barbie doll is created; boyfriend Ken appears in 1961.

1960   The United States has 85 million television sets; Great
        Britain 10.5 million; West Germany 2 million; France 1.5
        million.

        The Many Loves of Dobie Gillis premieres on television.

        The Food and Drug Administration approves the female
        oral contraceptive pill; by 1967, nearly 13 million women
        in the world will be using it.

        About one-half million unmarried couples are living
        together.

        The United States learns *The Twist* from Chubby Checker.

1961   The United States enters the Vietnam War, which will last
        until 1975.

1962   Helen Gurley Brown publishes the best-selling *Sex and the Single Girl.*

The first video games appear in the United States.

Marilyn Monroe dies of a drug overdose at age 36.

Silicone breast implants become available.

1963   The Beatles debut in England.

Feminist Betty Friedan publishes *The Feminine Mystique.*

1964   The Beatles' *I Want to Hold Your Hand* is an international hit and launches the British Invasion of rock stars to the United States.

The oldest baby boomers enter college.

Indiana Governor Matthew Welsh attempts to ban the Kingsmen hit *Louie, Louie* because he feels that it contains obscene material. After review by the FCC, the agency determines that the song's lyrics are indecipherable.

1965   The U.S. Supreme Court rules, in *Griswold v. State of Connecticut,* that laws prohibiting the use of birth control are unconstitutional.

The Pawnbroker becomes the first major Hollywood film to feature frontal nudity.

The Dating Game debuts on television.

1966   The National Organization for Women (NOW) is founded by Betty Friedan and other delegates to the Third National Conference of the Commission on the Status of Women.

The first sex change operation is performed at Johns Hopkins University.

Margaret Sanger dies at age 86.

1966, cont.   William Masters and Virginia Johnson publish *Human Sexual Response.*

      Georgie Girl becomes the first film to carry the label "recommended for mature audiences."

1967   *Rolling Stone* magazine debuts.

      Colorado legalizes abortion for cases of rape, fetal deformity, or risk to the woman's physical or mental health.

1968   The Women's Equality Action League is created.

      The oldest baby boomers graduate from college.

      The movie industry establishes the G, PG, R, and X rating system.

      Approximately 200 million television sets exist in the world.

      Alex Comfort publishes *The Joy of Sex.*

      The Grateful Dead introduce Americans to psychedelic rock.

      Burt Reynolds becomes first nude male portrait in *Cosmopolitan* magazine.

1969   The Internet is created when the Advanced Research Projects Agency connects four computers located at Stanford Research Institute, the University of California at Los Angeles, the University of Southern California, and the University of Utah.

      Woodstock Music and Art Fair is held in New York; an estimated one-half million people attend the three-day event.

      Midnight Cowboy becomes the first major X-rated film.

1970   Kate Millett publishes *Sexual Politics.*

The first CDs (compact discs) are manufactured in the United States.

William Masters and Virginia Johnson publish *Human Sexual Inadequacy.*

1972   The U.S. Senate approves the Equal Rights Amendment and sends it to the states for ratification.

The first issue of *Ms.* magazine is published.

HBO debuts on cable television.

1973   The Supreme Court rules in *Roe v. Wade* that a woman has a constitutional right to abortion.

Robert Sorenson publishes *Adolescent Sexuality in Contemporary America.*

The American Psychiatric Association removes homosexuality from its official diagnostic manual of mental illness.

The Supreme Court rules that a film may be banned if it is "patently offensive" to "average persons applying contemporary community standards."

1974   The Dalkon Shield Intrauterine Device (IUD) is found to be defective and dangerous and is withdrawn from the market.

Punk rock debuts in England.

Skateboarding is introduced.

1975   Bill Gates and Paul Allen start Microsoft.

Saturday Night Live debuts on network television.

Rap and hip-hop music are introduced in New York City, popularized by such artists as the Beastie Boys and Public Enemy.

1976   Shere Hite publishes *The Hite Report* on women's sexuality.

1977   The film *Saturday Night Fever* showcases disco music.

        Nintendo begins to produce computer games.

1978   More than 1 million unwed adolescent females become pregnant.

1979   The Sony Walkman is invented.

1981   The first cases of Acquired Immunodeficiency Syndrome (AIDS) are reported in New York.

        MTV debuts with 24-hour broadcasts.

1982   In June, the Equal Rights Amendment expires, three states short of ratification.

        Carol Gilligan publishes *In a Different Voice: Psychological Theory and Women's Development*, a landmark book on female morality.

1983   The Today Contraceptive Sponge, a female birth control device, is approved by the Food and Drug Administration.

1984   The number of divorces in the United States declines for the first time in two decades.

        Madonna releases her album *Like a Virgin*, which becomes a best-seller.

1985   Congress allocates $70 million for AIDS research.
        Almost 2 million unmarried couples cohabit, an increase of more than 300 percent from the previous decade.

        Michael Jackson releases his album *Thriller*, which becomes one of the most popular albums ever recorded.

1986   Japan introduces the *Game Boy* computer play system.

1987   One-half of all households in the United States have cable television.

1988   The cervical cap, a female contraceptive, is approved by the Food and Drug Administration.

About 95 percent of U.S. homes have at least one television set.

1989   In *Webster v. Reproductive Health Services*, the U.S. Supreme Court upholds laws limiting a woman's right to abortion.

The Recording Industry Association of America (RIAA) releases its universal parental warning sticker in early March that reads, "Explicit Lyrics—Parental Warning."

The Teenage Mutant Ninja Turtles characters are introduced.

1990   The Food and Drug Administration approves Norplant, a long-acting, reversible female hormonal contraceptive.

The 1968 X rating for films is replaced by NC-17 (no children under 17).

Linguistics expert Deborah Tannen publishes *You Just Don't Understand*, a groundbreaking book exploring gender differences in communication.

Missouri legislators introduce a bill in January that forbids the sale of records containing lyrics that are considered violent, sexually explicit, or perverse. Similar measures are introduced in twenty other states.

Rollerblading becomes popular.

1991   The United States enters the Persian Gulf War.

Worldwide, 10 million people are estimated to be HIV-positive, including 1 million in the United States.

Grunge music becomes popular.

1992   The Food and Drug Administration approves Depo-Provera, an injectable female hormonal contraceptive.

Americans spend $12 billion to buy or rent videotapes.

1993   The number of estimated worldwide AIDS cases rises to 2.5 million.

1994   The female condom is approved by the Food and Drug Administration.

About one-third of all American homes have computers.

1995   The Centers for Disease Control announces that in the United States, AIDS has become the leading cause of death for those between the ages of 25 and 44.

Monica Lewinsky reportedly begins an intimate relationship with President Bill Clinton.

The Today Contraceptive Sponge is taken off the market due to production problems. Introduced in 1983, the sponge was the largest-selling over-the-counter female contraceptive in the United States.

1996   About 45 million Internet users exist worldwide, including 30 million in the United States.

1997   The United Nations/AIDS Project reports that 30 million people are infected with HIV/AIDS.

1998   The Food and Drug Administration approves Viagra, a medication to alleviate erectile dysfunction.

1999   The World Health Organization (WHO) estimates that AIDS has caused the life expectancy in southern Africa to drop from 59 years in the early 1990s to 45 years after 2005.

The state of Vermont votes to enact into law a bill recognizing civil unions between gay or lesbian couples. Civil union, a legal institution parallel to marriage, grants the same rights and benefits to same-sex couples as married couples.

Michigan passes legislation aimed at creating a concert ratings system that is similar to the system used to rate movies.

2000   The Food and Drug Administration approves RU-486, a drug which has been in use in France and other parts of Europe since the late 1980s. RU-486, also known as Mifepristone, is a drug that induces spontaneous abortion when administered within the first seven weeks of pregnancy and followed by the drug Misoprostol.

The U.S. government spends $6.9 billion on AIDS/HIV treatment this year.

The Food and Drug Administration approves Lunelle, a monthly combined hormone injectable female contraceptive.

During this year, 5.1 billion e-mails are sent in the United States; 8.2 billion are sent worldwide.

The Federal Trade Commission (FTC) recommends that the music industry enforce FTC policies about underage purchase of CDs bearing stickered warnings regarding content and that the music industry cease advertising in media that have a "substantial" youth audience.

2001   The World Health Organization (WHO) estimates that around the world in 2001, there have been 3 million deaths from AIDS, including 2.3 million in sub-Saharan Africa. There are also 5 million new infections, bringing the total to 40 million infected worldwide, and Africa has the most people infected (more than 16 million), followed by south and southeast Asia (more than 6 million).

The Food and Drug Administration approves two new combined hormone female contraceptives, the vaginal ring (NuvaRing) and the contraceptive patch (Ortho Evra).

2001, Approximately one-half of all Americans use the Internet.
cont.

2002 The World Health Organization reports that women, for the first time, comprise 50 percent of the 42 million people living with AIDS worldwide.

About 80 percent of American children have access to computers at home or school.

The U.S. Drug Enforcement Agency (DEA) estimates that more than 8 million people have used the club drug Ecstasy at least once during their lifetimes.

MTV reportedly reaches 250 million homes worldwide.

Reality television programs such as *ElimiDate* and *Temptation Island* become increasingly popular among teens and adults alike.

2003 The United Nations/AIDS Project estimates that 40 million persons worldwide are living with HIV/AIDS.

Despite early promise, an experimental vaccine called AIDSVAX fails to shield users against HIV/AIDS infection, although some protection was experienced by a small number of African Americans who participated in the trial study. The vaccine was developed by VaxGen of California, which spent $200 million in research and production costs.

The Today Contraceptive Sponge is made available to the public again after having been withdrawn from the market in 1995 due to production problems.

The Food and Drug Administration approves the anti-HIV drug Fuzeon, a new class of medications called fusion inhibitors. Fusion inhibitors work by helping to block the HIV virus from entering the immune system cells that it ultimately destroys.

5

Biographical Sketches

The primary intent of this chapter is to introduce some of the major contributors to the study of dating and sexual behavior. The chapter focuses on key people and how they have increased people's understanding of the issues and problems presented in chapter 2, including such areas as character development and values, media influences on teenagers, teenage pregnancy, and sexuality education. These contributors are recognized leaders in their fields and represent such disciplines as psychology, sociology, marriage and family, adolescent development, human sexuality, parent education, and gender studies. They have made their contributions as educators, authors, consultants, analysts, theorists, therapists, laboratory researchers, and public speakers. Their various publications appear at the end of the chapter.

Bordo, Susan R.

Susan R. Bordo (1947–) is professor of English and women's studies and holds the Otis A. Singletary Chair in the humanities at the University of Kentucky. She lectures nationally on contemporary culture and the body, featuring topics such as beauty and attraction, body image, sexual coercion, and the impact of contemporary media. The inclusion of such topics in chapter 2 of this book makes Bordo's research especially applicable to the study of dating and sexuality.

Bordo's best-selling book, *Unbearable Weight: Feminism, Western Culture, and the Body* (1995) was the first of its kind to draw attention to the profound role of cultural images in the spread of eating disorders across race and class. Bordo seeks to raise consciousness of how female oppression works through cultural institutions. Her book is widely cited, discussed, and anthologized and is used in courses throughout the disciplines. Named a 1993 Notable Book by the *New York Times*, it was nominated for a Pulitzer Prize and received a Distinguished Publication Award from the Association for Women in Psychology.

Bordo's 1999 book, *The Male Body: A New Look at Men in Public and in Private*, also met with critical acclaim. The book details how men's (and women's) ideas about men's bodies are heavily influenced by society's expectations. Bordo offers a powerful cultural analysis of the male body, society's perceptions of maleness, male beauty standards, and sexual harassment.

Brooks-Gunn, Jeanne

Jeanne Brooks-Gunn is a researcher specializing in the physical and sexual developments that occur during adolescence. She also specializes in research focusing on family and community influences upon the development of children and teenagers, most notably designing and evaluating interventions to upgrade the well being of youngsters living in poverty and associated conditions.

Brooks-Gunn received her master's degree from Harvard University in 1970 and completed her doctoral studies at the University of Pennsylvania in 1975. She is currently the Virginia and Leonard Marx Professor of Child Development and Education at Teachers College, Columbia University. Brooks-Gunn is also the codirector of the Institute for Child and Family Policy at Columbia.

Brooks-Gunn has received numerous honors and distinctions throughout her professional career. In 1998, she received the Vice President's National Performance Review Hammer Award for her participation in the Federal Interagency Forum on Child and Family Statistics of the National Institute for Child Health and Human Development Research Network. She was also awarded the 1997 Nicholas Hobbs Award from the American Psychological Association's Division of Children, Youth, and Families for her contributions to policy research for youngsters. Brooks-Gunn also received the 1996 John B. Hill Award from the Society for Research on Adolescence for her lifetime contribution to research on adolescence. Brooks-Gunn has also served as past president of the Society for Research on Adolescence and is a Fellow in the American Psychological Association and the American Psychological Society.

Brooks-Gunn is the author and editor of more than 300 published articles and 15 books. Her books include *Consequences of Growing Up Poor* (Duncan and Brooks-Gunn, 1999); *Transitions through Adolescence: Interpersonal Domains and Context* (Graber, Brooks-Gunn, and Petersen, 1996); *Adolescent Mothers in Later Life* (Furstenberg, Morgan, and Brooks-Gunn, 1989); *Girls at Puberty: Biological and Psychosocial Perspectives* (Brooks-Gunn and Petersen, 1983); and *Encyclopedia of Adolescence* (Lerner, Petersen, and Brooks-Gunn, 1991). She also serves as an editor for Harvard University Press, specializing in books on youth and policy research in the United States.

Calderone, Mary S.

Mary S. Calderone (1904–1998) is recognized internationally as one of the early pioneers in the field of human sexuality education. She grew up in New York and received a medical degree from the University of Rochester in 1939. In the early 1950s, Calderone became medical director of the Planned Parenthood Federation of America, and shortly thereafter she began writing and speaking about birth control, family planning, and sexuality education.

In 1964, Calderone co-founded the Sexuality Information and Education Council of the United States (SIECUS), an organization designed to promote research, discussion, and education on the topic of human sexuality. The development and distribution of sex education materials for children and teenagers was among the more important institutional goals of SIECUS. Calderone remained executive director of SIECUS until 1975 and then served as its president from 1975 through 1982.

Calderone taught human sexuality at New York University from 1982 to 1988. She received many awards and commendations throughout her career, including a Lifetime Achievement Award from the Schlesinger Library, Radcliff/Harvard Universities; the Browning Award for Prevention of Diseases, American Public Health Association; the Margaret Sanger Award from the Planned Parenthood Federation of America; and the Elizabeth Blackwell Award for Distinguished Services to Humanity. Calderone also received twelve honorary doctorates over her career from such institutions as Columbia, Adelphi, Bucknell, and Hofstra Universities.

Among Calderone's more notable books are the *Manual of Family Planning and Contraceptive Practice* (1977), *The Family Book about Sexuality* (Calderone and Johnson, 1989), and *Talking with*

Your Child about Sex: Questions and Answers for Children from Birth to Puberty (Calderone and Ramey, 1982). Calderone died in 1998.

Cherlin, Andrew J.

Andrew J. Cherlin is a professor in the Sociology Department at Johns Hopkins University. He earned his undergraduate degree from Yale University in 1970 and completed his doctoral studies in sociology at the University of California, Los Angeles, in 1976. He is considered an expert in the fields of public policy, family studies, divorce, and remarriage and has published extensively in these areas.

In his 1992 book *Marriage, Divorce, and Remarriage,* Cherlin provides readers with a comprehensive examination of marriage dissolution, including demographic trends, explanations for divorce rates, consequences of separation, and racial as well as class implications. In *Public and Private Lives* (2001), he explores the larger social structures in which family relations are embedded and the activities of private life such as dating, courtship, and cohabitation.

In 1989–1990 Cherlin was Chair of the Family Section of the American Sociological Association, and in 1999, he was president of the Population Association of America. Cherlin is a recipient of a MERIT (Method to Extend Research in Time) Award from the National Institutes of Health for his research on the effects of family structure on children.

Coles, Robert

Robert Coles is a research psychiatrist for Harvard University Health Services and a professor of psychiatry and medical humanities at the Harvard Medical School. Coles received his undergraduate degree from Harvard University and earned his medical degree from Columbia University College of Physicians and Surgeons. He is best known for his explorations of children's and adolescents' lives and for books that explore their morality and character development. Coles's biography is included in this chapter because of the emphasis he places on moral reasoning and character. Sound moral character, he holds, has many implications for dating and sexual relationships, including the nurturance of sensible and sensitive styles of loving, mutual sensitivity and reciprocity, and responsible sexual decision making.

Coles is also the James Agee Professor of Social Ethics at Harvard University. He has taught courses at Harvard University, Harvard Medical School, Harvard Business School, Harvard Law School, the Harvard School of Education, and Harvard Extension School. He has been a visiting professor at Duke University in the history department for many years and is a founding member of the Center for Documentary Studies at Duke University.

Since 1961, Coles has published more than 1,300 articles, reviews, and essays in newspapers, magazines, journals, and anthologies. In books such as *The Spiritual Life of Children* (1991) and *The Moral Intelligence of Children* (1997), Coles describes how children and teens can be taught to become "smart" in their inner spiritual realm—to learn empathy, respect for themselves and others, and how to live the Golden Rule—through witnessing the conduct and caring of others and through moral conversations. Most of his books are based on a method of long-term direct observation and are expressed in his research subjects' narratives.

Coles has received numerous awards, including the Ralph Waldo Emerson Prize of Phi Beta Kappa (1967); the Anisfield-Wolf Award in Race Relations of the *Saturday Review* (1968); the Hofheimer Award of the American Psychiatric Association (1968); the McAlpin Medal of the National Association of Mental Health (1972); the Weatherford Prize of Berea College and the Council of the Southern Mountains (1973); the Lillian Smith Award of the Southern Regional Council (1973); the Pulitzer Prize (1973); and the John D. and Catharine MacArthur Foundation Fellowship Award (1981).

DeLamater, John D.

John D. DeLamater, professor of sociology at the University of Wisconsin, Madison, received his education at the University of California—Santa Barbara and the University of Michigan. He created the Human Sexuality course at the University of Wisconsin in 1975 and has taught it regularly since then. His research and writing are focused on social and psychological influences on human sexuality; his recent work is in the areas of HIV / AIDS and STD prevention. He is the author of many articles for various human sexuality and sociology research journals.

DeLamater is a Fellow of the Society for the Scientific Study of Sexuality and editor of the *Journal of Sex Research*. He has received numerous awards for excellence in teaching from the Department of Sociology and Interfraternity Council, Panhellenic Association and is a member of the Teaching Academy at the University of Wisconsin. He regularly teaches a seminar for graduate students on teaching undergraduate courses.

Donnerstein, Edward

Edward Donnerstein is professor of psychology, the director of the Center for Communication and Social Policy, and dean of social sciences at the University of California, Santa Barbara. He earned his doctorate in psychology in 1972. Prior to his appointment at the University of California, he taught at the University of Wisconsin.

Donnerstein is widely known for his contributions to the study of mass media violence, as well as media policy. He is particularly interested in the effects the mass media have on children and adolescents. He has published more than 180 scientific articles in all of these areas, and he serves on the editorial boards of a number of academic journals in both psychology and communication. He was a member of the American Psychological Association's (APA) Commission on Violence and Youth and the APA Task Force on Television and Society.

Donnerstein has testified at numerous governmental hearings, both in the United States and abroad, regarding the effects and policy implications surrounding mass media violence and pornography, including testimony before the U.S. Senate on TV violence. He has also served as a member of the U.S. Surgeon General's Panel on Pornography and the National Academy of Sciences Subpanel on Child Pornography and Child Abuse.

Elias, Maurice J.

Maurice J. Elias is a professor of psychology at Rutgers University, a member of the Leadership Team of the Collaborative for the Advancement of Social and Emotional Learning, a nationally recognized expert on child and parent problem solving, and a writer and contributor to numerous professional publications. At Rutgers, he specializes in clinical/community and school psychology and child, adolescent, and family development. He is licensed for professional psychology practice in New Jersey.

His numerous books focus on the complex dynamics of parenthood and what parents can do to foster healthy development in their offspring. The importance he places on good communication skills and mutual respect are important issues to consider when exploring adolescent dating and socialization in general. In the book *Emotionally Intelligent Parenting: How to Raise a Self-Disciplined, Responsible, and Socially Skilled Child* (Elias, Tobias and Friedlander, 2000), Elias breaks the mold of traditional parenting books by taking into account the strong role of emotions—those of parents and children—in psychological development. Elias details how to communicate with children on a deeper, more gratifying level and how to help them successfully navigate the intricacies of relating to others.

Elias's book *Raising Emotionally Intelligent Teenagers: Guiding the Way for Compassionate, Committed, and Courageous Adults* (Elias, Tobias, and Friedlander, 2002) sheds considerable light on adolescent challenges, such as issues concerning identity, self-confidence, peer pressure, dating and sexuality, responsibility, and individuation. The book has been translated into eight international editions, including translations into Spanish and Hebrew.

Erikson, Erik H.

Erik H. Erikson (1902–1994) was born in Frankfurt, Germany, and was one of the world's foremost psychoanalytic scholars. After finishing high school, Erikson visited various parts of Europe to study art. During one of his journeys, he was given an opportunity to study child analysis at the Vienna Psychoanalytic Institute. It was at this institute, under the guidance of Anna Freud, among others, that Erikson launched a brilliant career in the field of developmental psychology.

Erikson is most famous for creating a personality development theory that extends across the entire life cycle. Unlike Sigmund Freud, who placed emphasis on psychosexual stages of development, Erikson stressed psychosocial development throughout life. At each stage of development, he theorized, from birth to old age, there is a psychosocial crisis that must be resolved, eight crises in all. Harmonious personality development, he said, is characterized by the successful resolution of these psychosocial crises.

Erikson holds that adolescents are in the midst of resolving the crisis of Identity vs. Role Confusion. Erikson suggests that adolescents are confronted not only with issues related to their personal identities but that they must also grapple with an assortment of adult roles and responsibilities. How these forces interact will influence the course of psychosocial development, most notably one's interactions with others.

Once this identity crisis is resolved during the teenage years, Erikson proposes that young adults are motivated to fuse this newly established identity with those of others. This becomes apparent in the stage of Intimacy vs. Isolation. Although most young adults seek to gratify the need for intimacy through marriage or another long-term, committed relationship, nonsexual intimate relationships are also possible. Individuals may develop strong bonds of intimacy in friendships that offer, among other features, mutuality, empathy, and reciprocity.

Erikson's stages of Identity vs. Role Confusion and Intimacy vs. Isolation, then, are important to the study of dating and sexuality. From an Eriksonian perspective, maturity is likely among those who have achieved a sense of identity and are motivated to share themselves with others on a meaningful basis. Mature partners demonstrate comfort with who they are, as well as a capacity to share and understand. They are able to effectively communicate with one another and are sensitive and tolerant of each other's needs. Erikson recognizes that the growth of commitment, love, and devotion is much more prominent among highly mature people than among the immature.

Freud, Sigmund

Sigmund Freud (1856–1939) was an Austrian physician who forged a revolutionary theory of personality in which sexual motivation played a dominant role. Born in what is now Czechoslovakia, Freud received a medical degree from the University of Vienna in 1881. While practicing medicine in clinics, he spent considerable time seeking to understand abnormal brain functions and mental disorders, a pursuit that would eventually bring him to the fields of psychiatry and psychology.

Gradually, through treating neurotic patients with such techniques as hypnosis and free association (asking the patient to say spontaneously whatever comes into his or her mind), Freud became convinced that sexual conflict was the cause of most neuroses. Freud traced such conflict to the forces of sexual and aggressive urges and the clashes of these forces with the codes of conduct required by society.

Eventually, Freud developed psychoanalytic theory, which proposes, among other things, that one's past plays an important role in determining one's present behavior through psychosexual stages. Fundamental to Freud's theory are the notions that behavior is unconsciously motivated and that neuroses often have their origins in early childhood experiences that have subsequently become repressed. Freud also suggested that sexual urges were responsible for most human motivations. He held that because sexual thoughts and needs were often repressed, they were likely to provide unconscious motivation. Freudians would look to these unconscious motivations to explain the dating and sexual behaviors of adolescents.

Although many of Freud's views are controversial, many researchers in the fields of dating and human sexuality have been influenced by his theory of psychosexual development. According to this theory, the development and maturation of sexual and other body parts has great impact on early life experiences. Critics of psychoanalytic theory claim that many of Freud's concepts cannot be scientifically measured and are based on poor methodology. Some argue that his theories were bound to nineteenth-century Vienna and, furthermore, that he downplayed female sexuality. Proponents, however, point out how Freud's ideas have extended into many disciplines including history, literature, philosophy, and the arts. They contend that however one views Freud's specific theories, one cannot deny the power of his intellect and the strength of his motivation to discover new dimensions of human behavior.

Fromm, Erich

Erich Fromm (1900–1980) was a noted psychoanalytic scholar who explored the nature of productive and nonproductive facets of behavior within interpersonal relationships, including expressions of love. Fromm trained at the Berlin Psychoanalytic Institute and received his Ph.D. in psychology from the University of Heidelberg in 1922. He held teaching positions at Columbia University, Yale University, New York University, and Michigan State University.

Fromm maintained that men and women sometimes tend to alienate themselves and demonstrate hostile and aggressive forms of behavior. Fromm concentrated his energies on studying such negative behavior, particularly ways to overcome it. His works are directed toward the protection of humanity, including the need for people to unite with others and to feel like part of a group, such as within a family, church, or nation. Fromm saw control as a necessary way of life, including the setting of limits through boundaries, rules, and regulations.

In his writings, Fromm often stressed the importance of relating to others in a loving, caring fashion. He stressed the importance of altruistic love and proposed that loving should be an act of giving rather than receiving. He contended that love should embrace such elements as respect, concern, and understanding.

Furstenberg, Frank F., Jr.

Frank F. Furstenberg Jr. is a widely recognized authority in the fields of dating, human sexuality, and family studies research. He is the Zellerbach Family Professor of Sociology and a research associate in the Population Studies Center at the University of Pennsylvania. Furstenberg completed his undergraduate degree at Haverford College in Pennsylvania in 1961 and earned his doctoral degree in 1967 from Columbia University.

Furstenberg has published numerous books and research articles on teenage sexuality, pregnancy, and childbearing as well as on divorce, remarriage, and stepparenting. Among his more notable books are *Managing to Make It: Urban Families and Adolescent Success* (Furstenberg et al. 2000); *Divided Families: What Happens to Children When Parents Part* (Furstenberg and Cherlin, 1991); *Adolescent Mothers in Later Life* (Furstenberg, Morgan, and Brooks-Gunn, 1989); and *Teenage Sexuality, Pregnancy, and Childbearing* (Furstenberg, Menken, and Lincoln, 1981).

His current research projects focus on the family in the context of disadvantaged urban neighborhoods, adolescent sexual behavior, cross-national research on children's well being, urban education, and the transition from adolescence to adulthood. He is the Chair of the MacArthur Foundation Research Network on the Transition to Adulthood. In October 1966, he was made a member of the Institute of Medicine of the National Academy of Science.

Galinsky, Ellen

Ellen Galinsky is co-founder and president of the Families and Work Institute, a Manhattan-based nonprofit center for research on the changing family, workplace, and community. She is a leading authority and an author of publications focusing on work and family life. She also taught for more than 20 years at the Bank Street College of Education.

Galinsky was born in Pittsburgh, Pennsylvania in 1942 and received a graduate degree from the Bank Street College of Education in 1970. She is the author of sixteen books, including the 1981 *Between Generations: The Six Stages of Parenthood*, which explores the developmental dynamics of parenthood, particularly how it unfolds through a series of predictable stages. Galinsky feels that these stages bring a progressive transformation of parental self-images. Galinsky says that parents' self-images—not to mention parental development—are shaped by interactions with their children. Put another way, a child's development leads the parent from one stage to the next.

Another noteworthy book by Galinsky is *Ask the Children: The Breakthrough Study that Reveals How to Succeed at Work and Parenting* (2000). This book contains the results of Galinsky's comprehensive study that asked children and their parents for their views on work and family life. Galinsky discusses guilt-inducing myths often associated with working families, shares stories of how some of her subject families stay close, and outlines a set of operating principles to navigate work/family challenges.

Gelles, Richard J.

Richard J. Gelles is an internationally known expert on all forms of family violence, as well as on abusive dating relationships and acquaintance rape. He is currently Chair of the Child Welfare and Family Violence Program in the School of Social Work at the University of Pennsylvania. Gelles received his undergraduate degree from Bates College (1968), a master's degree in sociology from the University of Rochester (1971), and a Ph.D. in sociology from the University of New Hampshire (1973).

Gelles is the author or coauthor of twenty-one books and more than 100 articles and chapters on family violence. His 1997 book *Intimate Violence in Families* paints a sobering portrait of hidden victims of familial violence—siblings, parents, and the elderly—as well as an examination of violence within gay and lesbian couples. He also explores emotional and psychological abuse, sexual abuse, neglect, and abandonment. Gelles informs readers what is known about intervention and treatment program effectiveness, with special attention paid to intensive family preservation programs and men's treatment programs. In an earlier book, *International Perspectives on Family Violence* (Gelles and Cornell, 1991), Gelles offers a world view of domestic abuse, in the process offering convincing evidence that battering is a universal social problem.

Gelles is a member of the National Academy of Science's Panel on Assessing Family Violence Interventions. He also served as vice president for publications for the National Council on Family Relations. From 1973 to 1981, Gelles edited the journal *Teaching Sociology* and earned the Outstanding Contributions to Teaching Award in 1979 from the American Sociological Association. Gelles has presented innumerable lectures to family studies organizations, policy-making groups, and media groups.

Gilligan, Carol

Carol Gilligan is recognized as a leading contributor to the study of adolescence, moral reasoning, and women's development. Gilligan's insight into female moral development is particularly useful in a study of dating and sexuality, especially the manner in which values and attitudes shape the course of intimate relationships.

Born in 1936 in New York City, Gilligan received a master's degree in clinical psychology from Radcliffe University in 1960 and a doctorate degree in social psychology from Harvard University in 1964. Gilligan spent most of her teaching career at Harvard University and worked alongside such world-renowned psychologists as Erik Erikson and Lawrence Kohlberg (biographical sketches on both men are included in this chapter). It was with Kohlberg that Gilligan's interest in female morality began. Kohlberg had created a developmental approach to the study of morality in the 1970s, a stage theory suggesting that morality followed a sequential and predictable course. However, because Kohlberg's research was based exclusively on a male population, Gilligan extended his research to females. Gilligan also maintained that men are more apt to think in terms of rules and justice in their moral decision making and that women are more inclined to think in terms of caring and the relationships involved. Her ongoing research exploring a lifespan perspective of female moral development succeeded in opening a new chapter in the discipline of gender studies, and her theory is widely used and referred to by social scientists.

During her tenure at Harvard, Gilligan initiated and steered the Women's Psychology and Girls' Development Project, as well as the Project on Women's Psychology, Boys' Development, and the Culture of Manhood. In 1992, Gilligan received the prestigious Grawemeyer Award in Education, and in 1996 she was named one of *Time* magazine's twenty-five most influential people in the nation. In 1997, she received the Heinz Award for knowledge of the human condition and for her challenges to previously held assumptions in the field of human development. Following a distinguished 35-year career at Harvard, Gilligan accepted a full-time professorship at New York University.

Gilligan has authored and coauthored numerous books and publications. In addition to the critically acclaimed *In a Different Voice* (1983), Gilligan is the author of *The Birth of Pleasure* (2002). She is also the coauthor of *Women's Psychology and Girls' Development* (Brown and Gilligan, 1998), and *Between Voice and Silence: Women and Girls, Race and Relationship* (Taylor and Gilligan, 1997).

Gordon, Sol

Sol Gordon is one of the nation's most recognizable sexuality educators. As an author and speaker, he is renowned for his insight, humor, and honest approach to communication about sexuality, family studies, and relationships. Gordon received his B.A. and M.S. from the University of Illinois and his Ph.D. in psychology from the University of London (1953). Upon his retirement from Syracuse University, he was a Fellow of the APA and a member of the National Council on Family Relations and the American Association of Sex Educators, Counselors, and Therapists.

Gordon served as chief psychologist at the Philadelphia Child Guidance Clinic and the Middlesex County Mental Health Clinic. Gordon taught at Yeshiva University (1965–1969) and Syracuse University, where he was professor of child and family studies and founding director of the Institute for Family Research and Education (1970–1985). Dr. Gordon is a professor emeritus at Syracuse University, with a distinguished career as a clinical psychologist and sex educator, and he is the recipient of many scholarly awards.

He has written more than 100 articles for professional publications and has written numerous books. One of his most popular is *Raising a Child Responsibly in a Sexually Permissive World* (2000), which he wrote with his late wife Judith. In this book, the Gordons stress that children who are knowledgeable about sex are less vulnerable to being exploited and are less likely to exploit others. Gordon has lectured in every state of the United States as well as internationally in Australia, Japan, Sweden, Denmark, England, Israel, Germany, Thailand, New Zealand, and Holland.

Haffner, Debra W.

Debra W. Haffner served as executive director of the Sexuality Information and Education Council of the United States (SIECUS) between 1988–2000 and is considered one of the nation's leading authorities on sexuality and AIDS education. Haffner, who received a Bachelor of Arts degree in political science from Wesleyan University and a master's degree in public health from Yale School of Medicine, has written many articles and books on sexuality education and is responsible for designing and implementing a number of school and community sexuality education projects. During her tenure at SIECUS, Haffner raised more than $15 million for the organization, grew the budget more than sixfold, opened professional offices in New York City and Washington D.C., and increased the number of foundations who are supporting SIECUS from one to the current twenty-one.

Under Haffner's leadership, SIECUS created the HIV Prevention Program, the National Coalition to Support Sexuality Education, the Public Policy Program, the Community Advocacy Project, the International Initiative, the Outreach Initiative, the National Commission on Adolescent Sexual Health, the Internet Clearinghouse, the Religion Initiative, the Mid-Life and Older Adults Initiative, and the Media Program. Haffner has provided training on sexuality education to more than 13,000 people and spoken to more than 30,000 professionals.

In 1991, Haffner convened a National Guidelines Task Force of leading health, education, and sexuality professionals to develop the *Guidelines for Comprehensive Sexuality Education, Kindergarten–12th Grade* (1991). The *Guidelines* represented the first national model for comprehensive sexuality education. Since they were first published in 1991, the *Guidelines* have become the most widely recognized and implemented framework for comprehensive sexuality education in the country. More than 40,000 copies have been distributed in the United States alone. The *Guidelines* have also spread internationally. SIECUS has worked with organizations in Brazil, Nigeria, Russia, the Czech Republic, and Iceland on adapting *Guidelines* for these countries.

Among Haffner's other books are *From Diapers to Dating: A Parent's Guide to Raising Sexually Healthy Children* (2000) and *Beyond the Big Talk: Every Parent's Guide to Raising Sexually Healthy Teens—From Middle School to High School and Beyond* (2002). She has been honored by many organizations, including the Society for the Scientific Study of Sexuality, the Society of Public Health Education, the Society for Adolescent Medicine, the Robert Wood Johnson Medical School, and the Child Welfare League of America.

Hetherington, E. Mavis

E. Mavis Hetherington was a professor of psychology for many years at the University of Virginia until she retired in 1999. She earned her Ph.D. in psychology at the University of California at Berkeley. Hetherington is a past president of the Developmental Psychology Division of the American Psychological Association and of the Society for Research in Child Development in Adolescence. She has written and edited many books in the areas of child and adolescent development and has contributed dozens of articles to professional research journals.

Hetherington is well known for her work on the effects of divorce, one-parent families, and remarriage on children's development. Her book *For Better or for Worse: Divorce Reconsidered* (Hetherington and Kelly, 2002) provides readers with an in-depth investigation of marital dissolution and its effects on children. The book summarizes findings from the Virginia Longitudinal Study of Divorce, which analyzed how children and their families adapted to divorce over the course of time. Hetherington's longitudinal study followed an initial group of seventy-two children of divorce and their families as the parents began remarrying, becoming stepparents, and, in some cases, getting divorced once again.

From this long-term perspective, Hetherington identifies distinct pathways into and out of divorce and identifies kinds of marriages that predispose a couple to divorce and others that do not. She shows how women and girls experience divorce differently from men and boys; why single mother-son relationships and stepfather-daughter relationships are often difficult; why divorce presents a greater risk to adolescent children; and how mentoring and authoritative parenting can provide the needed buffering against the negative effects of divorce.

Hyde, Janet S.

Janet S. Hyde, professor and Chair of the Department of Psychology and Evjue-Bascom Professor of Women's Studies at the University of Wisconsin, Madison, received her education at Oberlin College and the University of California, Berkeley. She has taught a course in human sexuality since 1974, first at Bowling Green State University, then at Denison University, and now at the University of Wisconsin. Her research interests are in human sexuality, gender differences, and gender role development in children and teenagers.

Hyde is the author of the best-selling *Understanding Human Sexuality* (2003), which examines the science and psychology of the discipline while providing important information on such topics as contraception, safer sex, and sexually transmitted diseases. Hyde is also the author of *Half the Human Experience: The Psychology of Women* (1996), which offers a detailed and multicultural analysis of gender issues in the world today.

Hyde is currently president of the Society for the Scientific Study of Sexuality and is a Fellow of the American Psychological Association. She has received many other honors, including an award for excellence in teaching at Bowling Green State University, the Chancellor's Award for teaching at the University of Wisconsin, and the Kinsey Award from the Society for the Scientific Study of Sexuality for career contributions to sex research.

Kinsey, Alfred C.

Alfred C. Kinsey (1894–1956) ranks as one of the most influential human sexuality researchers in the United States. He was born in Hoboken, New Jersey, and received his Ph.D. in biology from Harvard in 1920. He became an instructor in biology at Indiana University shortly thereafter, and earned academic recognition for his work in the field of taxonomy (the science of identifying, naming, and classifying organisms). He remained on the faculty at Indiana University until his death in 1956.

Kinsey launched his detailed investigation of human sexual behavior in 1938. Over a span of 10 years, Kinsey and his staff interviewed more than 11,000 individuals (about 5,300 males and 5,900 females) using a sex history questionnaire that contained 521 items. The subjects represented a cross-section of geographical location, education, occupation, socioeconomic level, age, and religion in the United States. However, only white male and white female respondents were included in the published findings. This was because Kinsey deemed the population sample of black respondents insufficient in size for making analyses comparable to those made for whites.

In 1948, the research team of Kinsey and his Indiana University associates Wardell Pomeroy and Clyde Martin published *Sexual Behavior in the Human Male.* In 1953, Kinsey worked with Pomeroy, Martin, and Paul Gebhard to publish *Sexual Behavior in the Human Female.* These four researchers were chiefly responsible for the thousands of interviews conducted, with Kinsey himself handling more than 7,000 of them. This is a staggering total when one realizes that the average interview required between one and one-half to two hours of time.

Never before had a strictly scientific investigation like this aroused so much interest, not only among fellow researchers but among the general public as well. When the findings were released, prevailing conceptions of many facets of human sexuality were radically altered. Indeed, most readers of the Kinsey studies were astonished to discover how widespread certain sexual activities were in the United States. For example, most men and almost one-half of the women reported that they had engaged in premarital sex. Many couples also engaged in sexual practices considered objectionable by society at the time, such as oral sex. About 50 percent of married men and approximately 25 percent of married women also reported having had at least one extramarital affair.

Kinsey's research marked a major breakthrough in social science research. Although critics pointed to several research flaws (e.g., using a disproportionate number of uneducated males and too many college-educated females; interviewing only those subjects who were willing to disclose their sex lives), Kinsey's research had many positive dimensions. In addition to its magnitude and scope, an outstanding feature of Kinsey's research was the scholarly objectivity and sophisticated interviewing techniques Kinsey's staff used during the duration of the project. Due to Alfred Kinsey and his team, human sexuality research began to emerge as a legitimate and respectable branch of social science inquiry.

Kohlberg, Lawrence

Lawrence Kohlberg (1927–1987) was a psychologist and leading figure in the field of moral development. Kohlberg was born and raised in Bronxville, New York. After serving in the Merchant Marine following his high school graduation, Kohlberg enrolled in college and received a B.A. in 1949 and a Ph.D. in 1958 from the University of Chicago. Kohlberg taught at the University of Chicago from 1962 to 1968 and then became a full professor at Harvard University, a post he held until his death. He wrote many books and research articles, and he was the recipient of many awards and citations.

Kohlberg is widely recognized for his contributions to the study of the development of morality. Inspired by Swiss psychologist Jean Piaget's thoughts on morality, Kohlberg provided a more detailed structure in formulating a theory of moral development. Kohlberg felt that morality develops through a series of progressive, age-related stages. Like Piaget, Kohlberg viewed cognitive development as the foundation for moral thinking and reasoning.

Kohlberg believed that the successive moralities of children result from the cognitive restructuring of their experiences, not from a set of graded lessons taught by adults. Kohlberg also maintained that interrelatedness exists between the various stages. Kohlberg suggested that moral development is characterized by increasing differentiation and that each stage includes everything that took place at previous stages. Kohlberg outlined moral distinctions for each stage that a child had been only dimly aware of at a previous stage, and he organized them into a more adequate and comprehensive structure. He suggested that principles learned during early stages are either permanently buried or are selectively utilized, depending on one's level of cognitive development. Kohlberg's theory has application to the study of dating and sexuality, particularly the manner in which values shape the course of intimate relationships. Kohlberg's work also stimulated the work of Carol Gilligan (see her biographical sketch in this chapter), who revised his theory so that it captured female moral development.

Maccoby, Eleanor E.

Eleanor E. Maccoby is an international authority on the development of children's social behavior, particularly as it relates to family functioning and parental child-rearing methods. Her work has pointed to the differences in the social development of boys and girls, although it has also illuminated many ways in which they are similar. Before joining the Stanford faculty in 1958 and after receiving her Ph.D. from the University of Michigan in 1950, Maccoby taught at Harvard University.

Maccoby has been widely published in research journals and has written a number of authoritative books in the fields of child and adolescent psychology. The book *Adolescents after Divorce* (Buchanan, Maccoby, and Dornbusch, 2000) traces teenagers from 1,100 divorcing families to discover what factors account for healthy adjustment. *The Two Sexes: Growing Up Apart, Coming Together* (1999) offers readers a thought-provoking analysis of how individuals express their sexual identity at successive periods of their lives, a topic she had begun to work on earlier in her career in the book *The Psychology of Sex Differences* (Maccoby and Jacklin, 1994).

Maccoby has been the recipient of many honors and awards throughout her distinguished career. For example, she was the recipient of the 1988 Distinguished Scientific Contribution Award (APA), the 1996 American Psychological Foundation Gold Medal Award for Lifetime Achievements in the Science of Psychology, and the 1987 Award for Distinguished Scientific Contributions to Child Development (Society for Research in Child Development).

Maslow, Abraham H.

Abraham H. Maslow (1908–1970) was instrumental in shaping humanistic theory, a school of thought in psychology that emphasizes an individual's uniqueness, personal potential, and inner drives. Born in Brooklyn, New York, Maslow earned his B.A., M.A., and Ph.D. from the University of Wisconsin. From 1935 to 1937, Maslow taught at Columbia University on a Carnegie Fellowship, and he later taught at Brooklyn College. Following his stay at Brooklyn, Maslow went to Brandeis University, where he became chairman of the Department of Psychology. He remained at Brandeis until his death in 1970.

Among his accomplishments, Maslow served as president of the American Psychological Association in 1967. He was also president of the Massachusetts Psychological Association and chairman of the Personality and Social Psychology Division of the American Psychological Association. Maslow also was the founder of the *Journal of Humanistic Psychology*.

Maslow earned critical acclaim with his theory of self-actualization, which distinguished between an organism's basic needs, such as the need for food, water, sex, security, and companionship, and what Maslow called metaneeds. The basic needs are often called deficiency needs because the organism is motivated toward fulfilling some deficiency. Maslow contended that only after these more basic needs are met can a person move on toward meeting metaneeds such as those for beauty, justice, and goodness. The ability to meet these higher needs, Maslow held, can lead to happiness, satisfaction, and, possibly, self-actualization.

Maslow's concept of self-actualization has application to the study of dating and sexual relationships. Self-actualized partners are making full use of their talents and abilities in life and are able to engage in relationships that are authentic and meaningful. Such a relationship itself offers a climate of comfort and security as well as a vehicle for the exchange of belongingness and love. Moreover, constructive feedback between partners creates an atmosphere of trust and authenticity, important ingredients of self-actualization.

Masters, William H. and Johnson, Virginia A.

William H. Masters (1915–) and Virginia E. Johnson (1925–) are perhaps the most famous team of investigators in the history of human sexuality research. Masters received his M.D. degree from the Rochester School of Medicine in 1943. At Washington University in St. Louis, Masters began exploring the physiology of sex, as well as the treatment of sexual dysfunction. Spurred on by the generally favorable response to Alfred Kinsey's human sexuality research, Masters decided to launch a more detailed investigation on sexual functioning and enlisted the services of research associate Virginia Johnson, who had studied psychology and sociology at Missouri University. Masters and Johnson, who later married and then divorced, began a laboratory physiological study of human sexual response in 1957. The two founded, and served as codirectors of, the Masters and Johnson Institute in St. Louis. Their laboratory research would eventually yield significant contributions to the field of human sexuality research: *Human Sexual Response* (1966), *Human Sexual Inadequacy* (1970), and *Sex and Human Loving* (1988).

Unlike Kinsey, Masters and Johnson directly and systematically observed (and filmed) sexual intercourse and self-stimulation, or masturbation. Whereas Kinsey's research represented a statistical analysis of sexual behavior, Masters and Johnson broke new ground by using sophisticated instrumentation to measure the physiology of sexual response. They recruited a total of 694 participants of both genders for laboratory study (all were paid for their services), including 276 married couples. The unmarried subjects participated primarily in noncoital research activities, such as studies of ejaculatory processes in men or of the ways in which different contraceptive devices affected female sexual responses. Although most subjects were between the ages of 18 and 40, Masters and Johnson included a group of subjects over the age of 50 in order to study the effects of aging on sexual response. A careful screening procedure was designed to weed out exhibitionists and people with emotional disturbances.

Following a tour of Masters and Johnson's laboratory facilities and inspection of the equipment to be used in the studies, each subject was invited to a private practice session. The purpose of this was to accustom people to engaging in sexual activity in a laboratory environment. When actual experimental sessions began, subjects performed acts of masturbation or sexual intercourse while being filmed or wearing devices that recorded physiological response to sexual stimulation. For example, a subject might wear electrode terminals connected to an electrocardiograph that would produce a record of his or her heart's activity during sexual intercourse. Or a subject might have a band placed around his penis to record size and speed of erection in response to manual stimulation.

In more than 10,000 sessions, Masters and Johnson recorded subjects' responses to sexual stimulation and discovered striking similarities between the responses of men and women. From this research, Masters and Johnson developed a sexual model of response called the sexual response cycle. The model consists of four stages of physiological response during which two basic physiological reactions occur: an increased concentration of blood in bodily tissues in the genitals and female breasts, and increased energy in the nerves and muscles throughout the body.

The Masters and Johnson research model was not without its critics. For example, many viewed the laboratory setting as dehumanizing and mechanizing sex. Many critics felt that the emphasis placed on the physiology of sex downplayed its interpersonal and emotional aspects. Some objected to the research design on ethical grounds, claiming the project was an invasion of privacy. Finally, critics wondered if Masters and Johnson had selected a representative sample of the population. In fact, most of the subjects were well educated and more affluent than the average person. Moreover, their willingness to perform sexually under laboratory conditions suggested that they were not typical. Overall, though, the research of Masters and Johnson had enormous impact on the field of human sexuality. For the first time, scientific evidence on the physiology of the orgasmic response was systematically gathered. Because of these efforts, laboratory studies of sexual arousal began to achieve a new level of respectability among scientific researchers.

Parke, Ross D.

Ross D. Parke is an expert in the field of family studies and has made many research contributions in the areas of parent-child relations, fatherhood, child and adolescent development, and abusive relationships. He is distinguished professor of psychology and director of the Center for Family Studies at the University of California, Riverside. He is a past president of the Developmental Psychology Division of the American Psychological Association, and is currently editor of the *Journal of Family Psychology*. Parke is a graduate of the University of Waterloo in Ontario, Canada, having completed his doctoral studies in 1965.

Parke's recent examinations of fatherhood have received critical acclaim in psychological and sociological circles. In *Fatherhood* (1996) he explores how men enact their fatherhood in a variety of ways in response to their particular social and cultural circumstances. In *Throwaway Dads* (Parke and Brott, 1999), Parke reveals how humans as a society have wittingly and unwittingly built nearly insurmountable barriers that restrict men's involvement with their children and families. He explodes the myths of neglectful, uninterested, abusive, deadbeat, and lazy fathers with real-life studies and statistics. Parke also offers proposals for steps that men, women, employers, the medical community, the media, and the government can take to promote men's involvement in their children's lives.

His current research focuses on the development of social behavior in young children. He is examining mother-father differences in styles of interaction and examining the linkages that exist between family and peer social systems. Parke is interested in the lessons that are learned in the family that, in turn, influence children's adaptation to peers.

Pipher, Mary

Mary Pipher is a clinical psychologist and an adjunct clinical professor at the University of Nebraska. She completed an undergraduate degree in cultural anthropology from the University of California at Berkeley in 1969 and earned her doctoral degree from the University of Nebraska in 1977. Pipher's teaching and literary contributions combine her training in the fields of psychology and anthropology. Her special area of interest is how American culture affects the mental health of its people, particularly women. Her research on women in general, and female teenagers in particular, makes her writings especially applicable to this text. In addition to her teaching contributions, Pipher travels the country sharing her ideas with community groups, schools, and healthcare professionals.

The most well known of Pipher's works is her 1995 best-selling *Reviving Ophelia: Saving the Selves of Adolescent Girls*. This book reached the number one position on the *New York Times* best-seller list and remained on the overall list for 154 weeks. In this book, Pipher maintains that Americans live in a looks-obsessed, sexist, "girl-poisoning" culture, and despite the advances of feminism, she feels that girls continue to struggle to find their true, inner selves. Pipher blends her writing with painfully honest case histories to illustrate the struggles required of adolescent girls to maintain a true sense of self. Pipher believes that many young teenagers lose spark, interest, and even IQ points as society forces a choice between being shunned for staying true to oneself and struggling to stay within a narrow definition of femininity. Pipher offers concrete suggestions for ways by which girls can build and maintain a strong sense of self.

Pollack, William S.

William S. Pollack is a clinical psychologist and is the codirector of the Center for Men at McLean Hospital, Harvard Medical School. He is also an assistant clinical professor of psychiatry at the Harvard Medical School, and is a founding member and Fellow of the Society for Psychological Study of Men and Masculinity of the American Psychological Association. Pollack's research is useful because it helps in better understanding male behavior as it relates to dating and sexual interactions.

An internationally recognized authority on boys and men, Pollack is founder and director of the Real Boys Educational Programs.

The programs are designed to free boys from rigid, traditional gender roles. The programs give practical advice to parents, teachers, counselors, coaches, and others about how to raise boys today and cover such topics as sibling wars, aggressive behavior at school, dealing with death or divorce, and exposure to violent television shows and video games.

Pollack is the author of several best-selling books, including *Real Boys' Voices* (2001) and *Real Boys: Rescuing Our Sons from the Myths of Boyhood* (1999). The books explore how many boys often appear tough, confident, and cheerful but are often sad, lonely, and confused. Pollack shows how society's mixed messages to boys put them at risk for maladjustment and unnecessary anxiety. He sheds light on the inner emotional experiences of boys and tells readers how society needs to improve how it raises, teaches, and relates to its boys. In an earlier book, *In a Time of Fallen Heroes* (Pollack and Betcher, 1995), Pollack expounds upon the nature of each male's internal struggles, victories, and losses in a search for the sense of manhood.

Sanger, Margaret

Margaret Sanger (1883–1966) initiated and led the movement to find safe and effective methods of birth control. She became interested in women's health issues through her experiences in nursing. Sanger worked with many poor women in New York for whom pregnancy was a "chronic condition" and who often induced their own abortions, frequently dying in the process.

Frustrated in her efforts to help these women through medical channels, Sanger left nursing and founded the National Birth Control League in 1914. Although the league's magazine, *Woman Rebel*, did not violate the Comstock Act of 1873 (which made it illegal to send contraceptive information through the mail), other birth control publications that she helped circulate did. Sanger barely escaped imprisonment by fleeing to Europe, where she visited birth control clinics in London.

Sanger returned to the United States in 1915; and in 1916, she opened a birth control clinic in Brooklyn where women could obtain diaphragms and birth control information, including the publication *Birth Control Review*. Because New York law forbade the distribution of contraceptive information, she was jailed for thirty days and the clinic was closed. But ultimately she won the right to keep the clinic open, and within two years, doctors were legally allowed to dispense contraceptive information.

Sanger began the American Birth Control League in 1921, and she promoted the concepts of women's health and reproductive rights both at home and abroad. Sanger also promoted birth control research, fighting for a reliable birth control method that could be controlled by women, but it was not until 1960 that birth control pills became available in the United States.

Schwartz, Pepper

Pepper Schwartz is a sociologist specializing in intimate relationships, human sexuality, and family studies. Schwartz was born in 1945 in Chicago, Illinois, and earned a master's degree from Washington University in 1968. She completed her doctoral studies at Yale University in 1974 before launching a teaching career at the University of Washington in Seattle. She has taught there for more than thirty years.

Schwartz is past president of the Society for the Study of Sexuality and a charter member of the International Academy of Sex Research. She has written or cowritten twelve books, writes several magazine and Web columns, and also appears on Lifetime Television. She is the coauthor of *The Gender of Sexuality* (Schwartz and Rutter, 1998), a book that examines how and why sexual behavior and issues are different for women and men. She also coauthored the highly successful *American Couples* (Blumstein and Schwartz, 1985), which explored relational dynamics and the interplay that exists with such areas as finances, household decision making, sexual intimacy, and children.

In her book *Ten Talks Parents Must Have with Their Children about Sex and Character* (Schwartz and Cappello, 2000), Schwartz writes that it is more important than ever for parents and their children to communicate openly about these vital issues. The book offers parents advice on what to say to their children not just about sex, but about safety, character, peer pressure, ethics, meeting people on the Internet, and mixed messages from TV. The book also helps parents to clarify their own values while providing creative tools to enhance communication.

Steinberg, Laurence D.

Laurence D. Steinberg is considered an expert in the field of adolescent growth and development. He graduated from Vassar College in 1974 and received his Ph.D. in human development and family studies from Cornell University in 1977. Steinberg is a Fellow of the American Psychological Association's Division of Developmental Psychology and is currently the president of the Society for Research on Adolescence. He has taught previously at the University of California, Irvine, and the University of Wisconsin, Madison.

Steinberg is the author of numerous scholarly articles on adolescent development as well as numerous books capturing the interplay that exists between parent and teenager. In *You and Your Adolescent: A Parent's Guide for Ages 10–20* (Steinberg and Levine, 1997), Steinberg offers advice on such topics as physical health, psychological development, and socialization skills. In his book *Crossing Paths: How Your Child's Adolescence Triggers Your Own Crisis* (1994), Steinberg examines the profound impact teenagers have on their parents and shares how confusion and conflict are as common for parents as for teenagers. Steinberg explores the emotional turmoil that a child's adolescence can initiate in parents and recommends practical ways to avoid or lessen stress levels among all concerned.

Tannen, Deborah

Deborah Tannen is one of the nation's leading experts on gender differences in communication style and relationship dynamics. Tannen holds an undergraduate degree from Harpur College (since renamed Binghamton University) in 1966 and two master's degrees, one in English literature from Wayne State University in 1970 and one in linguistics from the University of California at Berkeley in 1976. She earned a doctoral degree in linguistics from the University of California at Berkeley in 1979.

Tannen is on the linguistics department faculty at Georgetown University, where she is a full professor. She has also taught at Princeton University and was a Fellow at the Center for Advanced Study in the Behavioral Sciences in Palo Alto, California. She has published nineteen books and nearly 100 articles on gender differences in communication style and has been awarded five honorary doctorates. Her research has wide application to the study of dating relationships and the complex dynamics attached to sexual intimacy.

Tannen is best known for her book *You Just Don't Understand: Women and Men in Conversations* (1990), which brought gender differences in communication style to the forefront of public awareness. Her book *Talking from 9 to 5: Women and Men at Work*

(2001) explains women's and men's conversational rituals and the language barriers they unintentionally erect in the business world. Her latest book, *I Only Say This because I Love You: Talking to Your Parents, Partner, Sibs, and Kids When You're All Adults* (2002), discusses why talking to family members about sensitive subjects such as loss or sibling rivalry is so often painful and problematic even when all those involved are adults.

In addition to her college teaching responsibilities, Tannen has lectured all over the world. Her audiences have included corporations; professional societies such as the American Psychological Association and the National Council on Family Relations; and college faculty, administrators, and trustees. Combining the results of years of research and observation with videotaped real-life footage of conversational styles, Tannen supplies her audiences a new framework for understanding what happens in conversations both in the workplace and at home.

Tannen is a frequent guest on television and radio news and information shows. She has appeared on such television programs as *20/20, 48 Hours, CBS News, ABC's World News Tonight,* and *Good Morning America.* She has been featured in major magazines and newspapers including *Newsweek, Time,* the *New York Times,* the *Washington Post,* and the *Harvard Business Review.*

Wallerstein, Judith S.

Judith S. Wallerstein is considered one of the world's foremost authorities on the effects of divorce on children. Wallerstein attended Columbia University and the Topeka Institute for Psychoanalysis, and she received her Ph.D. in psychology at Lund University in Sweden. She is the founder and executive director of the Judith Wallerstein Center for the Family in Transition in Marin County, California. The Wallerstein Center conducts research and provides education and counseling for separated, divorced, or remarried families. Wallerstein has also taught at the School of Social Welfare and the School of Law at the University of California at Berkeley as well as at Kansas University and the Menninger School of Psychiatry.

Wallerstein is best known for her longitudinal research focusing on the long-term effects of divorce on children, which she translated into several successful books. Her book *Surviving the Breakup: How Children and Parents Cope with Divorce* (Wallerstein and Kelly, 1996) grew out of her California Children of Divorce

Study, launched in 1971. In the study, Wallerstein began studying a group of 131 children whose parents were all going through divorce. She tracked the youngsters from childhood, through their adolescent struggles, and eventually into adulthood. Her book *Second Chances: Men, Women, and Children a Decade after Divorce* (Blakeslee and Wallerstein, 1989), comprised the 10- and 15-year follow-up reports on her research.

Her book *The Unexpected Legacy of Divorce: A 25-Year Landmark Study* (Wallerstein, Blakeslee and Lewis, 2001), describes the feelings, expectations, and memories of divorce that these youngsters carried into adulthood and brought into their own intimate relationships. Wallerstein shares how adult children of divorce essentially view life differently from those not experiencing divorce.

Wallerstein also cowrote *The Good Marriage: How and Why Love Lasts* (Wallerstein and Blakeslee, 1996), based on her research between 1990 and 1991, examining fifty stable and fulfilling marriages. Wallerstein describes what she considers the four basic types of marriage: romantic, rescue, companionate, and traditional. She identifies the stages through which a marriage evolves and explains the nine psychological tasks—including separating from the family of origin and making a safe place for conflict—that must be undertaken by anyone committed to building a good marriage.

References

Blakeslee, Sandra, and Judith S. Wallerstein. 1989. *Second Chances: Men, Women, and Children a Decade after Divorce.* Boston: Houghton Mifflin.

Blumstein, Philip, and Pepper Schwartz. 1985. *American Couples.* New York: Pocket.

Bordo, Susan R. 1995. *Unbearable Weight: Feminism, Western Culture, and the Body.* San Diego, CA: University of California Press.

———. 1999. *The Male Body: A New Look at Men in Public and in Private.* New York: Farrar, Straus, and Giroux.

Brooks-Gunn, Jeanne, and Anne C. Petersen. 1983. *Girls at Puberty: Biological and Psychosocial Perspectives.* Scranton, PA: Perseus.

Brown, Lyn Mikel, and Carol Gilligan. 1998. *Women's Psychology and Girl's Development.* New York: Random House.

Buchanan, Christy M., Eleanor E. Maccoby, and Sanford M. Dornbusch.

2000. *Adolescents after Divorce*. Cambridge, MA: Harvard University Press.

Calderone, Mary. 1977. *Manual of Family Planning and Contraceptive Practice*. Melbourne, FL: Krieger.

Calderone, Mary, and Eric W. Johnson. 1989. *The Family Book about Sexuality (Rev. Ed.)*. New York: Harper and Row.

Calderone, Mary, and James W. Ramey. 1982. *Talking with Your Child about Sex: Questions and Answers for Children from Birth to Puberty*. New York: Random House.

Cherlin, Andrew J. 1992. *Marriage, Divorce, and Remarriage*. Cambridge, MA: Harvard University Press.

———. 2001. *Public and Private Lives: An Introduction*. New York: McGraw-Hill.

Coles, Robert. 1991. *The Spiritual Life of Children*. Boston: Houghton Mifflin.

———. 1997. *The Moral Intelligence of Children: How to Raise a Moral Child*. Boston: Houghton Mifflin.

Duncan, Greg J., and Jeanne Brooks-Gunn (Eds.). 1999. *Consequences of Growing Up Poor*. New York: Russell Sage Foundation.

Elias, Maurice J., Stephen E. Tobias, and Brian S. Friedlander. 2000. *Emotionally Intelligent Parenting: How to Raise a Self-Disciplined, Responsible, and Socially Skilled Child*. New York: Crown.

———. 2002. *Raising Emotionally Intelligent Teenagers: Guiding the Way for Compassionate, Committed, and Courageous Adults*. New York: Crown.

Furstenberg, Frank F., Jr., and Andrew J. Cherlin. 1991. *Divided Families: What Happens to Children When Parents Part*. Cambridge, MA: Harvard University Press.

Furstenberg, Frank F., Jr., Jane Menken, and Richard Lincoln (Eds.). 1981. *Teenage Sexuality, Pregnancy, and Childbearing*. Baltimore, MD: University of Pennsylvania Press.

Furstenberg, Frank F., Jr., Phillip S. Morgan, and Jeanne Brooks-Gunn. 1989. *Adolescent Mothers in Later Life*. Port Chester, NY: Cambridge University Press.

Furstenberg, Frank F., Jr., Thomas Cook, Jacquelynne Eccles, Glen Elder, Jr., and Arnold Sameroff. 2000. *Managing to Make It: Urban Families and Adolescent Success*. Chicago, IL: University of Chicago Press.

Galinsky, Ellen. 1981. *Between Generations: The Six Stages of Parenthood*. New York: Times.

————. 2000. *Ask the Children: The Breakthrough Study that Reveals How to Succeed at Work and Parenting.* Scranton, PA: HarperTrade.

Gelles, Richard J. 1997. *Intimate Violence in Families.* Thousand Oaks, CA: Sage.

Gelles, Richard J., and Claire Cornell. 1991. *International Perspectives on Family Violence.* New York: Free Press.

Gilligan, Carol. 1983. *In a Different Voice: Psychological Theory and Women's Development.* Cambridge, MA: Harvard University Press.

————. 2002. *The Birth of Pleasure.* New York: Alfred Knopf.

Gordon, Sol, and Judith Gordon. 2000. *Raising a Child Responsibly in a Sexually Permissive World.* Holbrook, MA: Adams Media.

Graber, Julia A., Jeanne Brooks-Gunn, and Anne C. Petersen (eds.). 1996. *Transitions through Adolescence: Interpersonal Domains and Context.* Mahwah, NJ: Lawrence Erlbaum.

Haffner, Debra W. 1991. *Guidelines for Comprehensive Sexuality Education, Kindergarten–12th Grade.* Washington, DC: Sexuality Information and Education Council of the United States.

————. 2000. *From Diapers to Dating: A Parent's Guide to Raising Sexually Healthy Children.* New York: Newmarket Press.

————. 2002. *Beyond the Big Talk: Every Parent's Guide to Raising Sexually Healthy Teens, from Middle School to High School and Beyond.* New York: Newmarket Press.

Hetherington, E. Mavis, and John Kelly. 2002. *For Better or for Worse: Divorce Reconsidered.* New York: Norton.

Hyde, Janet S. 1996. *Half the Human Experience: The Psychology of Women.* Boston: D. C. Heath.

————. 2003. *Understanding Human Sexuality (8th Ed.).* New York: McGraw-Hill.

Kinsey, Alfred C., Wardell B. Pomeroy, and Clyde E. Martin. 1948. *Sexual Behavior in the Human Male.* Philadelphia: Saunders.

Kinsey, Alfred C., Wardell B. Pomeroy, Clyde E. Martin, and Paul Gebhard. 1953. *Sexual Behavior in the Human Female.* Philadelphia: Saunders.

Lerner, Richard M., Anne C. Petersen, and Jeanne Brooks-Gunn (eds.). 1991. *Encyclopedia of Adolescence.* Bristol, PA: Taylor and Francis.

Maccoby, Eleanor E. 1999. *The Two Sexes: Growing Up Apart, Coming Together.* Cambridge, MA: Harvard University Press.

Maccoby, Eleanor E., and Carol J. Jacklin. 1994. *The Psychology of Sex Differences.* Stanford, CA: Stanford University Press.

Masters, William H., and Virginia Johnson. 1966. *Human Sexual Response.* Boston: Little, Brown.

———. 1970. *Human Sexual Inadequacy.* Boston: Little, Brown.

Masters, William H., Virginia Johnson, and Robert C. Kolodny. 1988. *Sex and Human Loving.* Boston: Little, Brown.

Parke, Ross. D. 1996. *Fatherhood.* Cambridge, MA: Harvard University Press.

Parke, Ross. D., and Armin Brott. 1999. *Throwaway Dads.* Boston: Houghton-Mifflin.

Pipher, Mary. 1995. *Reviving Ophelia: Saving the Selves of Adolescent Girls.* New York: Ballantine.

Pollack, William S. 1999. *Real Boys: Rescuing Our Sons from the Myths of Boyhood.* New York: Henry Holt.

———. 2001. *Real Boys' Voices.* New York: Penguin.

Pollack, William S., and William Betcher. 1995. *In a Time of Fallen Heroes.* New York: Guilford Press.

Schwartz, Pepper, and Dominic Cappello. 2000. *Ten Talks Parents Must Have with Their Children about Sex and Character.* Westport, CT: Hyperion.

Schwartz, Pepper, and Virginia Rutter. 1998. *The Gender of Sexuality.* Thousand Oaks, CA: Pine Forge.

Steinberg, Laurence D., and Anne Levine. 1997. *You and Your Adolescent: A Parent's Guide for Ages 10–20.* New York: HarperCollins.

Steinberg, Laurence, D., and Wendy Steinberg. 1994. *Crossing Paths: How Your Child's Adolescence Triggers Your Own Crisis.* New York: Simon and Schuster.

Tannen, Deborah. 1990. *You Just Don't Understand: Women and Men in Conversations.* New York: HarperCollins.

———. 2001. *Talking from 9 to 5: Women and Men at Work.* New York: HarperCollins.

———. 2002. *I Only Say This because I Love You: Talking to Your Parents, Partner, Sibs, and Kids When You're All Adults.* New York: Ballantine.

Taylor, Jill McLean, and Carol Gilligan. 1997. *Between Voice and Silence: Women and Girls, Race and Relationship.* Cambridge, MA: Harvard University Press.

Wallerstein, Judith S., and Joan B. Kelly. 1996. *Surviving the Breakup: How Children and Parents Cope with Divorce.* New York: Basic.

Wallerstein, Judith S., and Sandra Blakeslee. 1996. *The Good Marriage: How and Why Love Lasts.* New York: Warner.

Wallerstein, Judith S., Sandra Blakeslee, and Julia Lewis. 2001. *The Unexpected Legacy of Divorce: The 25-Year Landmark Study.* Westport, CT: Hyperion.

6

Facts and Data

This chapter is designed to present readers with important facts and data related to dating and sexuality. This meaningful, insightful, and applied information complements text throughout the book, especially the material discussed in Chapters 1 and 2. In some cases, the statistical portraits are used to summarize key points or provide a visual display when words alone cannot adequately describe a concept. The gathered figures and tables thus serve to offer a variation of text material, in the process providing readers with ways to better understand important concepts and, with visual aids, to better remember them.

Figure 6.1 U.S. Fertility Rate, 1910–2000

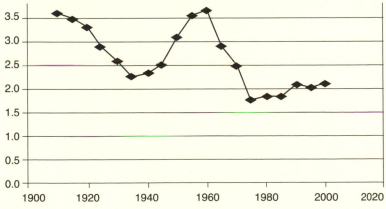

Source: U.S. Bureau of the Census. 2000. Current Population Reports, Series P20-537. *America's Families and Living Arrangements: March 2000.* Washington, DC: U.S. Government Printing Office.

Figure 6.2 Activities of U.S. Individuals Online, 2001
(Given as a Percentage of Internet Users)

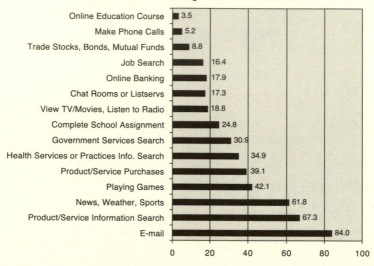

Source: U.S. Department of Commerce. 2002. *A Nation Online: How Americans Are Expanding Their Use of the Internet.* Washington, DC: Economics and Statistics Administration.

Figure 6.3 Internet Use among U.S. Children and Teenagers, 1998 and 2001
(Given as Percentages of the U.S. Population)

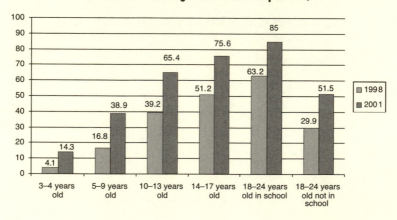

Source: U.S. Department of Commerce. 2002. *A Nation Online: How Americans Are Expanding Their Use of the Internet.* Washington, DC: Economics and Statistics Administration.

Figure 6.4 Major Internet Activities among Children and Teenagers, 2001

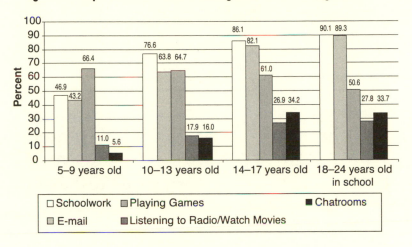

Source: U.S. Department of Commerce. 2002. *A Nation Online: How Americans Are Expanding Their Use of the Internet.* Washington, DC: Economics and Statistics Administration.

Figure 6.5 Sexual and Reproductive Timeline
Men and women experience important sexual and reproductive events at similar ages.

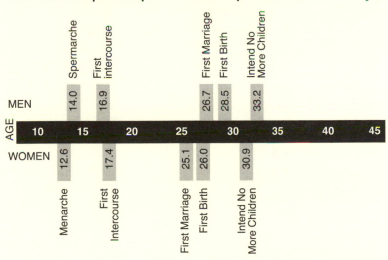

Source: Alan Guttmacher Institute. 2002. "Sexual and Reproductive Health," *Facts in Brief.* New York: Author.

Figure 6.6 Teen Pregnancy and Sexual Activity

Teen Pregnancy

U.S. teenagers have higher pregnancy rates, birthrates, and abortion rates than adolescents in other developed countries.

Teen Sexual Activity

Differences in levels of teenage sexual activity across developed countries are small.

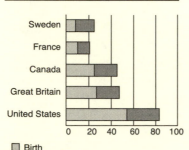

☐ Birth
■ Abortion
Rate per 1,000 women aged 15–19

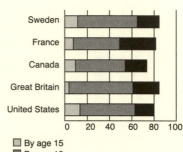

☐ By age 15
☐ By age 18
■ By age 20
% of women 20–24 who had sex in their teenage years

Source: Alan Guttmacher Institute. 2001. "Teenagers' Sexual and Reproductive Health," *Facts in Brief.* New York: Author.

Figure 6.7 Unmarried-Partner Households by Sex of Partners and Race and Hispanic Origin of Households: 2000

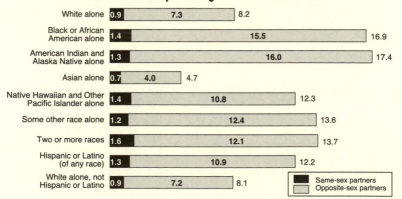

Notes: Percent same-sex partners and percent opposite-sex partners may not add to total percent unmarried-partner households because of rounding.
Percent of all coupled households. For information on confidentiality protection, non-sampling error and definitions, see www.census/prod/cen2000/docs/sf1.pdf

Source: U.S. Bureau of the Census. 2003. "Married-Couple and Unmarried-Partner Households." *Census 2000 Special Reports.* Washington, DC: U.S. Government Printing Office.

Figure 6.8 Households by Type, 1990 and 2000

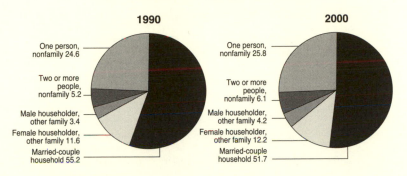

Note: Percent distribution. For information on confidentiality protection, nonsampling error, and definitions, see www.census.gov/prod/cen2000/doc/sf7.pdf

Source: U.S. Bureau of Census. 2003. "Married-Couple and Unmarried-Partner Households." *Census 2000 Special Reports*. Washington, DC: U.S. Government Printing Office.

Figure 6.9 Percent Change in Number of Jobs by Most Significant Source of Education or Training (Projected 2000–2010)

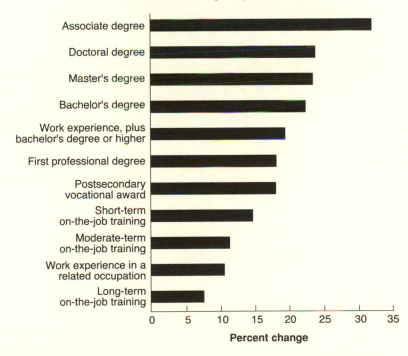

Source: U.S. Department of Labor. 2002. *Occupational Outlook Handbook, 2002–2003*. Washington, DC: U.S. Bureau of Labor Statistics.

Table 6.1
Major Types of Sexually Transmitted Diseases

STD Name	Category	Incidence*	Major Symptoms	Treatment
Chlamydia	Bacterial	3 million	Genital discharge: burning when urinating; sometimes no symptoms	Antibiotics
Human papilloma virus	Viral	5.5 million	Genital warts, raised and flat in appearance	No cure; some drugs may provide symptomatic relief or slow viral progression
Gonorrhea	Bacterial	650,000	Genital discharge; burning or itching during urination	Antibiotics
Hepatitis B	Viral	125,000	Chronic flu-like symptoms; jaundice; dark urine	No cure; some drugs may provide symptomatic relief or slow viral progression
Genital herpes	Viral	1 million	Itching, burning, or pain in the genital area; genital blisters or sores	No cure; some drugs may provide symptomatic relief or slow viral progression
HIV/AIDS	Viral	40,000	No symptoms may appear for years until symptoms of AIDS occur	No cure; some drugs may provide symptomatic relief or slow viral progression
Syphilis	Bacterial	70,000	Painless genital sores; rash 3–6 weeks after sores disappear	Antibiotics
Vaginitis ("Trich")	Bacterial	5 million	Itching, burning vaginal pain; abnormal vaginal discharge	Antibiotics

*Estimated number of new cases every year
Source: Adapted from Centers for Disease Control and Prevention. 2001. *Tracking the Hidden Epidemics: Trends in STDs in the United States.* Atlanta, GA: Author

Table 6.2
Median Ages at First Marriage, 1900–2000

Year	Men	Women
1900	25.9	21.9
1910	25.1	21.6
1920	24.6	21.2
1930	24.3	21.3
1940	24.3	21.5
1950	22.8	20.3
1960	22.8	20.3
1970	23.2	20.8
1980	24.7	22.0
1990	26.1	23.9
1993	26.5	24.5
1994	26.7	24.5
1995	26.9	24.5
1996	27.1	24.8
1997	26.8	25.0
1998	26.7	25.0
1999	26.9	25.1
2000	26.8	25.1

Source: U.S. Bureau of the Census. 2000. Current Population Reports, Series P20-537. *America's Families and Living Arrangements: March 2000.* Washington, DC: U.S. Government Printing Office.

Table 6.3
The Baby Boom in the United States, 1946–1964

Year	Number of Births in Millions	Year	Number of Births in Millions
1940	2,559	1968	3,502
1941	2,703	1969	3,606
1942	2,989	1970	3,731
1943	3,104	1971	3,556
1944	2,939	1972	3,258
1945	2,858	1973	3,137
1946	**3,411**	1974	3,160
1947	**3,817**	1975	3,144
1948	**3,637**	1976	3,168
1949	**3,649**	1977	3,327
1950	**3,632**	1978	3,333
1951	**3,823**	1979	3,494
1952	**3,913**	1980	3,612
1953	**3,965**	1981	3,629
1954	**4,078**	1982	3,681
1955	**4,097**	1983	3,639
1956	**4,218**	1984	3,669
1957	**4,300**	1985	3,761
1958	**4,255**	1986	3,757
1959	**4,245**	1987	3,809
1960	**4,258**	1988	3,910
1961	**4,268**	1989	4,041
1962	**4,167**	1990	4,158
1963	**4,098**	1991	4,111
1964	**4,027**	1992	4,065
1965	3,760	1993	4,000
1966	3,606	1994	3,979
1967	3,521		

Source: U.S. Bureau of the Census. 2000. Current Population Reports, Series P20-537. *America's Families and Living Arrangements: March 2000*. Washington, DC: U.S. Government Printing Office.

Table 6.4
Common Street Terms for Club Drugs

Street Term	Club Drug Definition
Banana split	Combination of 2C-B (Nexus) with other illicit substances, particularly LSD (Lysergic Acid Diethylamide)
Batmans	Methylenedioxymethamphetamine (MDMA)
Bean	A capsule containing drugs; MDMA (Methylenedioxymethamphetamine)
Bibs	MDMA (Methylenedioxymethamphetamine)
Boomers	Psilocybin/Psilocin; LSD
Bumping up	Methylenedioxymethamphetamine (MDMA) combined with powder Cocaine
Cafeteria-style use	Using a combination of different club drugs
Candy ravers	Young people who attend raves; rave attendees who wear candy jewelry
Caps	Heroin; Psilocybin/Psilocin; Crack; Gamma Hydroxybutyrate (GHB)
Charity	Methylenedioxymethamphetamine (MDMA)
Circles	Rohypnol
Dead road	Methylenedioxymethamphetamine (MDMA)
Doses	LSD
E	Ecstasy (Methylenedioxymethamphetamine; MDMA)
E-bombs	MDMA (Methylenedioxymethamphetamine)
E-puddle	Sleeping due to MDMA use/exhaustion
E-tard	Person under the influence of MDMA (Methylenedioxymethamphetamine)
Easy lay	Gamma Hydroxybutyrate (GHB)
Egyptians	Methylenedioxymethamphetamine (MDMA)
Exiticity	Methylenedioxymethamphetamine (MDMA)
Fantasy	Gamma Hydroxybutyrate (GHB)
Flipping	Methylenedioxymethamphetamine (MDMA)
Forget-me pill	Rohypnol
Four leaf clover	Methylenedioxymethamphetamine (MDMA)
Georgia home boy	Gamma Hydroxybutyrate (GHB)
Goop	Gamma Hydroxybutyrate (GHB)
GWM	Methylenedioxymethamphetamine (MDMA)
H-bomb	Ecstasy (MDMA) mixed with Heroin
Hammerheading	MDMA (Methylenedioxymethamphetamine) used in combination with Viagra
Happy drug	Methylenedioxymethamphetamine (MDMA)
Hugs and kisses	Combination of Methamphetamine and Methylenedioxymethamphetamine (MDMA)
Hype	Heroin addict; an addict; Methylenedioxymethamphetamine (MDMA)
Igloo	Methylenedioxymethamphetamine (MDMA)
Jellies	Depressants; MDMA in gel caps
Kitty flipping	Use of Ketamine and MDMA
Liquid ecstasy	Gamma Hydroxybutyrate (GHB)
Liquid X	Gamma Hydroxybutyrate (GHB)
Love flipping	Use of Mescaline and MDMA
Lovers' special	Methylenedioxymethamphetamine (MDMA)
Parachute down	Use of MDMA after Heroin
Party pack	Combination of 2C-B (Nexus) with other illicit drugs, particulary MDMA (Methylene-dioxymethamphetamine; Ecstasy)
Peeper(s)	MDMA user(s)
Piggybacking	Simultaneous injection of 2 drugs; sequential use of more than one methylene-dioxymethamphetamine (MDMA) tablet
Pikachu	Pills containing PCP and Ecstasy
Rave energy	Methylenedioxymethamphetamine (MDMA)
Rib	Rohypnol; Methylenedioxymethamphetamine (MDMA)
Ritual spirit	Methylenedioxymethamphetamine (MDMA)
Roach-2	Rohypnol
Scoop	Gamma Hydroxybutyrate (GHB)
Sextasy	Ecstasy used with Viagra
Sleep	Gamma Hydroxybutyrate (GHB)

Street Term	Club Drug Definition
Smurfs	Methylenedioxymethamphetamine (MDMA)
Snackies	Methylenedioxymethamphetamine (MDMA) adulterated with Mescaline
Soap	Gamma Hydroxybutyrate (GHB); Crack Cocaine; Methamphetamine
Somatomax	Gamma Hydroxybutyrate (GHB)
Speedies	Methylenedioxymethamphetamine (MDMA) adulterated with Amphetamine
Stacks	Methylenedioxymethamphetamine (MDMA) adulterated with Heroin or Crack
Super X	Combination of Methamphetamine and Methylenedioxymethamphetamine (MDMA)
Tabs	LSD; Methylenedioxymethamphetamine (MDMA)
Troll	Use of LSD and MDMA

Source: Adapted from Office of National Drug Control Policy. 2002. *Street Terms: Drugs and the Drug Trade.* Drug Policy Information Clearinghouse. Rockville, MD: Author.

Table 6.5
Major Birth Control Methods

Method	Category	How Used	Effectiveness	STD Prevention
Abstinence	Natural	Couple decides not to have coitus	Perfect*: 100% Typical**: 100%	100% reduced risk
Male condom	Barrier	Creates a barrier between penis & vagina	Perfect: 97% Typical: 84%	Latex condoms reduce STD risks
Female condom	Barrier	Creates a barrier between penis & vagina	Perfect: 95% Typical: 85%	Has not been extensively tested for STD prevention
Depo Provera	Hormonal	Prevents ovulation and implantation of fertilized egg	Perfect: 99% Typical: 99%	Does not reduce STD risks; using a male latex condom may reduce risk
Diaphragm Cervical Cap	Barrier	Provides cervical barrier; spermicide kills sperm	Perfect: 94% Typical: 84%	Spermicide somewhat reduces STD risks
Fertility Awareness	Natural	Couple abstains from coitus on fertile days	Perfect: 90% Typical: 80%	Does not reduce STD risks; using a male latex condom may reduce risk
IUD	Mechanical	Prevents implantation of fertilized egg	Perfect: 95% Typical: 95%	Does not reduce STD risks; using a male latex condom may reduce risk
Norplant	Hormonal	Prevents ovulation and implantation of fertilized egg	Perfect: 99% Typical: 99%	Does not reduce STD risks; using a male latex condom may reduce risk
Pill	Hormonal	Prevents ovulation and implantation of fertilized egg	Perfect: 99% Typical: 95%	Does not reduce STD risks; using a male latex condom may reduce risk
Spermicides	Chemical	Kills sperm	Perfect: 95% Typical: 77%	Spermicide somewhat reduces STD risks
Sterilization	Surgical	Prevents fertilization of egg by sperm	Perfect: 99% Typical: 99%	Does not reduce STD risks; using a male latex condom may reduce risk

*The method is used perfectly (exactly as directed and without fail)
**The method is not used exactly as directed or is not used every time
Source: Adapted from U.S. Department of Health and Human Services. 2000. *Your Contraceptive Choices for Now, for Later.* Washington, DC: Author.

Table 6.6
Cumulative AIDS Cases in the United States by Age, 2001

Age	Number of Cumulative AIDS Cases
Under 5	6,975
Ages 5 to 12	2,099
Ages 13 to 19	4,428
Ages 20 to 24	28,665
Ages 25 to 29	105,060
Ages 30 to 34	179,164
Ages 35 to 39	182,857
Ages 40 to 44	136,145
Ages 45 to 49	80,242
Ages 50 to 54	42,780
Ages 55 to 59	23,280
Ages 60 to 64	12,898
Ages 65 or older	11,555

Source: Centers for Disease Control and Prevention. 2002. National Center for HIV, STD, and TB Prevention. *HIV/AIDS Surveillance Report.* Atlanta, GA: Author.

Table 6.7
Cumulative AIDS Cases in the United States by Race/Ethnicity, 2001

Race or Ethnicity	Number of Cumulative AIDS Cases
White, not Hispanic	343,889
Black, not Hispanic	313,180
Hispanic	149,752
Asian/Pacific Islander	6,157
American Indian/Alaska Native	2,537
Race/ethnicity unknown	634

Source: Centers for Disease Control and Prevention. 2002. National Center for HIV, STD, and TB Prevention. *HIV/AIDS Surveillance Report.* Atlanta, GA: Author.

Table 6.8a
AIDS Cases in the United States by Exposure Category, 2001

Exposure Category	Male	Female	Total*
Men who have sex with men	368,971	—	368,971
Injecting drug users	145,750	55,576	201,326
Men who have sex with men and inject drugs	51,293	—	51,293
People with hemophilia/coagulation disorder	5,000	292	5,292
People who have heterosexual contact	32,735	57,396	90,131
Recipients of blood transfusion, blood components, or tissue	5,057	3,914	8,971
Risk factor not reported or identified	57,220	23,870	81,091

*Includes 3 persons whose sex is unknown.

Table 6.8b
AIDS Cases of Children* in the United States by Exposure Category

Exposure Category	Number of AIDS Cases
Hemophilia/coagulation disorder	236
Mother with or at risk for HIV infection	8,284
Receipt of blood transfusion, blood components, or tissue	381
Risk not reported or identified	173

*Persons under age 13 at the time of diagnosis.
Source: Centers for Disease Control and Prevention. 2002. National Center for HIV, STD, and TB Prevention.
HIV/AIDS Surveillance Report. Atlanta, GA: Author.

Table 6.9
U.S. States or Territories Reporting Most AIDS Cases, 2001

State/Territory	Number of Cumulative AIDS Cases
New York	149,341
California	123,819
Florida	85,324
Texas	56,730
New Jersey	43,824
Pennsylvania	26,369
Illinois	26,319
Puerto Rico	26,119
Georgia	24,559
Maryland	23,537

Source: Centers for Disease Control and Prevention. 2002. National Center for HIV, STD, and TB Prevention.
HIV/AIDS Surveillance Report. Atlanta, GA: Author.

Table 6.10
Married and Unmarried Partner Households by Metropolitan Residence Status: 2000
(For information on confidentiality protection, nonsampling error, and definitions, see www.censu.gov/prod/cen2000/dac/st1.pdf)

Household type and sex of householder	Total		In a metropolitan area				Not in a metropolitan area	
			In central city		Not in central city			
	Number	Percent of all households	Number	Percent of all households	Number	Percent of all households	Number	Percent of all households
Total households[1]	105,480,101	79.9	32,753,918	31.1	51,550,967	48.9	21,175,216	20.1
Total coupled households[2]	59,969,000	78.7	15,189,744	25.3	32,024,737	53.4	12,754,519	21.3
Married-couple households	54,493,232	78.5	13,232,903	24.3	29,525,090	54.2	11,735,239	21.5
Male householder	47,449,405	77.9	11,101,326	23.4	25,867,380	54.5	10,480,699	22.1
Female householder	7,043,827	82.2	2,131,577	30.3	3,667,710	51.9	1,254,540	17.8
Unmarried-partner households	5,475,768	81.4	1,958,841	36.7	2,499,647	45.6	1,019,280	18.6
Opposite-sex partners	4,881,377	80.9	1,709,317	35.0	2,240,426	45.9	931,634	19.1
Male householder	2,615,119	79.7	849,082	32.5	1,233,987	47.2	532,050	20.3
Female householder	2,266,258	82.4	860,235	38.0	1,006,439	44.4	399,584	17.6
Same-sex partners	594,391	85.3	247,524	41.6	259,221	43.6	87,646	14.7
Male householder	301,026	86.3	135,546	45.0	124,261	41.3	41,219	13.7
Female householder	293,365	84.2	111,978	38.2	134,960	46.0	46,427	15.8

[1]Total includes other types of households including family and nonfamily households which do not contain either spouses or unmarried partners.

[2]Coupled households represent the total of married-couple and unmarried-partner households.

Source: U.S. Bureau of the Census. 2003. "Married-Couple and Unmarried-Partner Households." Census 2000 Special Reports. Washington, DC: U.S. Government Printing Office.

7

Directory of Organizations, Associations, and Agencies

This chapter contains a comprehensive listing of organizations, associations, and agencies related to the study of dating and sexuality. The names and mailing addresses of these sources are included as well as their URLs and telephone numbers. For the dual purpose of convenience and organization, the presentation of these sources is organized according to the sequence of problems, controversies, and solutions presented in Chapter 2.

Dating and Sexual Values

Advocates for Youth
1025 Vermont Avenue NW, Suite 200
Washington, DC 20005
Telephone: 202-347-5700; Fax: 202-347-2263
http://www.advocatesforyouth.org/about/index.htm

Advocates for Youth creates programs and advocates for policies that help young people make informed and responsible decisions about their reproductive and sexual health. Advocates for Youth provides information, training, and strategic assistance to youth-serving organizations, policy makers, youth activists, and the media in the United States and the developing world. Programs include the promotion of responsible dating behaviors, comprehensive sexuality education, and the prevention of sexually transmitted diseases.

Center for the Advancement of Ethics and Character
605 Commonwealth Avenue
Boston, MA 02215
Telephone: 617-353-3262; Fax: 617-353-3924
http://www.bu.edu/education/caec/files/flash.htm

The Center for the Advancement of Ethics and Character serves as a resource for adults in their role as moral educators. It sponsors research initiatives and publications on moral and character education, and educates teachers who can provide students with an intellectual framework for discussing, understanding, and practicing core virtues. Located at Boston University, the center urges national dialogue on issues of moral education, thus helping adults to become more competent in the study of ethics and character.

Character Counts/Josephson Institute
4640 Admiralty Way, Suite 1001
Marina del Rey, CA 90292-6610
Telephone: 310-306-1868; Fax: 310-827-1864
http://www.charactercounts.org/

The purpose of the Character Counts/Josephson Institute is to fortify the lives of American young people with consensus ethical values called the "Six Pillars of Character." These values, which transcend divisions of race, creed, politics, gender, and wealth, are trustworthiness, respect, responsibility, fairness, caring, and citizenship. Sexual responsibility is also one of the program areas.

Center for the Fourth and Fifth Rs
SUNY Cortland
P.O. Box 2000
Cortland, NY 13045
Telephone: 607-753-2455; Fax: 607-753-5980
http://www.cortland.edu/www/c4n5rs

The Center for the Fourth and Fifth Rs (Respect and Responsibility) serves as a regional, state, and national resource in character education. A growing national movement, character education is essential to the task of building a moral society and developing schools that are civil and caring communities. The center disseminates articles on character education, sponsors an annual summer institute in character education, publishes a newsletter, and is building a network of schools committed to teaching respect, responsibility, and other core ethical values as the basis of good character.

Center for the Study of Ethical Development
206A Burton Hall
178 Pillsbury Drive SE
Minneapolis, MN 55455
Telephone: 612-624-0876
http://education.umn.edu/csed/

The Center for the Study of Ethical Development began in the early 1970s as faculty and students from various disciplines began to meet informally to discuss research on moral development. In 1982, the center was formally established under the direction of noted morality researcher James Rest. The center primarily undertakes moral judgment research and seeks to design and improve moral judgment research instruments.

Character Education Partnership
1025 Connecticut Avenue NW, Suite 1011
Washington, DC 20036
Telephone: 800-988-8081
http://www.character.org/

The Character Education Partnership (CEP) is a nonpartisan coalition of organizations and individuals dedicated to developing moral character and civic virtue in the nation's youth as one means of creating a more compassionate and responsible society. The center holds that core ethical values such as respect, responsibility, and honesty can be both a matter of consensus and a model for youth. Information on sexual values and decision making is available from the center.

Coalition for Positive Sexuality
P.O. Box 77212
Washington, DC 20013-7212
Telephone: 773-604-1654
http://www.positive.org/Home/index.html

The Coalition for Positive Sexuality (CPS) is a grassroots direct-action volunteer organization. The purpose of this coalition is twofold: first, to give teens the information they need to take care of themselves and in so doing affirm their decisions about sex, sexuality, and reproductive control; and second, to facilitate dialogue in and out of the public schools on condom availability and sex education.

Communitarian Network
2130 H Street NW, Suite 703
Washington, DC 20052
Telephone: 202-994-7997
http://www.gwu.edu/~ccps/

The Communitarian Network is a coalition of individuals and organizations engaged in moral and ethical issues and concerns. The Communitarian Network is a nonsectarian, nonpartisan, transnational association. The organization offers extensive resources and links, including information regarding sexual values and decision making.

Ethics Resource Center
1747 Pennsylvania Avenue NW, Suite 400
Washington, DC 20006
Telephone: 202-737-2258; Fax: 202-737-2227
http://www.ethics.org

The Ethics Resource Center (ERC) is dedicated to building a community that shares the common values of honesty, respect, trust, and excellence. The group feels that these values are fundamental to how people conduct their work as an organization, how they act as employees, and how they treat each other as individuals. The center seeks to develop ways to hold people responsible for practicing these values.

Jefferson Center for Character Education
P.O. Box 4137
Mission Viejo, CA 92690-4137
Telephone: 949-770-7602; Fax: 949-450-1100
http://www.jeffersoncenter.org/default.htm

The Jefferson Center for Character Education is a national, nonprofit, nonsectarian organization that addresses the need to teach character education in both public and private schools. Its mission is to produce and promote values education programs that cut across ethnic, cultural, and religious lines. Among the values taught by the center are honesty, respect, responsibility, integrity, and caring.

Media Impact on Dating and Sexuality

About Face
P.O. Box 77665
San Francisco, CA 94103-5133
Telephone: 415-436-0212
http://www.about-face.org

About Face is a nonprofit organization that seeks to remove negative and distorted images of women in the media as well as developing personal activism and media literacy around images of girls and women in the media. The organization's website contains excellent resource material, including media facts, research articles, books, and links to other important websites.

Action Coalition for Media Education (ACME)
6400 Wyoming Boulevard NE
Albuquerque, NM 87109
Telephone: 505-828-3377; Fax: 505-828-3142
http://www.acmecoalition.org/

Action Coalition for Media Education (ACME) is an organization representing the interests of educators, youth leaders, community organizers, parents, researchers, students, children, teens, schools/school districts, community and nonprofit organizations, and anyone else who advocates for media literacy education that inspires citizens to action on important issues. A particular emphasis is placed on critically examining the world of media and for people to become advocates for democratic media reform. In doing so, the organization feels that teenagers will have the opportunity to become active, engaged citizens and lifelong learners.

Action for Media Education
4756 University Village Place NE, Suite 310
Seattle, WA 98105
Telephone: 206-525-3035
http://www.action4mediaed.org/

Action for Media Education seeks to increase community awareness of the importance of media literacy. The organization provides support and training for media literacy education activities in schools, homes, organizations, agencies, and groups working with children and youth. This organization recognizes the importance of quality programming for viewers of all ages, as well as the promotion of positive role models and meaningful family interactions.

Alliance for a Media Literate America (AMLA)
721 Glencoe Street
Denver, CO 80220
Telephone: 888-775-2652
http://www.amlainfo.org/

The Alliance for a Media Literate America (AMLA) is committed to promoting media literacy education that is focused on critical inquiry, learning, and skill building rather than on media bashing and blame. This national, grassroots membership organization seeks to help in promoting better health, combating violence, removing stereotypes, helping young people develop important life skills, sparking important community discussions, and giving voice to creative expression. The AMLA promotes the adoption of media literacy education into public school curricula, including directing teachers and administrators to resources and training available to support their efforts and supporting and/or conducting research that will help states to adopt comprehensive media literacy standards.

Center for Media Education (CME)
2120 L Street NW, Suite 200
Washington, DC 20037
Telephone: 202-331-7833; Fax: 202-331-7841
http://www.cme.org/about.html

The Center for Media Education (CME) is a national nonprofit organization dedicated to creating a quality electronic media culture for children and youth, their families, and the community. Over the years, the CME has been active both in expanding children's educational television programming and in encouraging television and Internet safeguards for children and teens.

Center for Media Literacy
3101 Ocean Park Boulevard, Suite 200
Santa Monica, CA 90405

Telephone: 310-581-0260; Fax: 310-581-0270
http://www.medialit.org/

The Center for Media Literacy is a nonprofit organization that believes media literacy is a critical life skill for children and adults in today's media culture. This organization focuses on helping the general public to understand the messages conveyed through visual images (television and movies), music, and advertising. In addition, the center promotes the alliance of organizations with a vested interest in the education of children and adults, including community and religious organizations, educational institutions, government agencies, and private corporations.

Children Now
Children and the Media Program
1212 Broadway, Fifth Floor
Oakland, CA 94612
Telephone: 510-763-2444; Fax: 510-763-1974
http://www.childrennow.org/media/index.html

Children Now is a research and action organization dedicated to ensuring that children grow up in economically secure families and have quality health coverage; a positive media environment; a good early education; and safe, enriching after-school activities. The organization's Media Program works to improve the quality of news and entertainment media both for children and about children's issues, paying particular attention to media images of race, class, and gender. The Media Program seeks to accomplish its goals through media industry outreach, independent research, and public policy development.

Kaiser Family Foundation
Sex on TV
2400 Sand Hill Road
Menlo Park, CA 94025
Telephone: 650-854-9400; Fax: 650-854-4800
http://www.kff.org/content/archive/1458/

The Kaiser Family Foundation is a source of facts and analysis for policy makers, the media, the healthcare community, and the general public. On its website, the foundation examines both the amount and the nature of television's sexual messages, paying special attention to references to such issues as contraception, safer sex, and waiting to have sex. Attention is given to broadcast, public, cable, independent, and premium channels.

Media Watch
P.O. Box 618
Santa Cruz, CA 95061-0618
Telephone: 800-631-6355
http://www.mediawatch.com

Media Watch challenges abusive stereotypes and other biased images commonly found in the media, including those related to sexism and racism. Media Watch, which began in 1984, distributes educational videos, media literacy information, and newsletters to help create more informed consumers of the mass media. The organization believes that education will help create a more active citizenry who will take action against sexism, racism, and violence in the media.

National Institute on Media and the Family
606 Twenty-Fourth Avenue South, Suite 606
Minneapolis, MN 55454
Telephone: 612-672-5437; Fax: 612-672-4113
http://mediaandthefamily.org/index.shtml

The National Institute on Media and the Family is a national resource for research, education, and information about the impact of media on children and families. The National Institute on Media and the Family was created to provide information about media products and their likely impact on children to parents and other adults so they can make informed choices.

Teen Health and the Media
University of Washington
Experimental Education Unit
Box 357925
Seattle, WA 98195
Telephone: 206-543-9414
http://depts.washington.edu/thmedia/

The Teen Health and the Media website is a virtual meeting place for teens, parents, educators, health professionals, and others who share a strong commitment to teens' health. Through the vehicle of media literacy, the organization encourages young people to make healthy choices and to interact with the media both as critical viewers and as creators. The organization is based in the College of Education at the University of Washington.

University of Iowa Department of Communication Studies
Gender, Ethnicity, and Race in the Media
105 Becker Communication Studies Building
University of Iowa
Iowa City, IA 52242-1498
Telephone: 319-335-0575; Fax: 319-335-2930
http://www.uiowa.edu/~commstud/resources/index.html

The University of Iowa's Department of Communication Studies focuses on the different media, modes, and uses of communication that exist in the world to foster scholarly understanding in both undergraduate and graduate students. The website examines advertising, feminist media, gender and the media, minority portrayals, and sexual orientation.

Internet Romance and Sex

Center for Online Addiction
eBehavior, LLC
P.O. Box 72
Bradford, PA 16701
Telephone: 877-292-3737; Fax: 814-368-9560
http://www.netaddiction.com/index.htm

The Center for Online Addiction is a treatment clinic and training institute specializing in cyber-disorders such as cybersex addiction, cyberaffairs, problem day trading, compulsive online shopping and gambling, and childhood Internet addiction. This organization provides a range of professional services, including corporate seminars and healthcare training, that focus on cyber-wellness. The programs are designed to promote health and well being and to help individuals maximize their use of technology while retaining a balance in their lives.

Childnet International
Studio 14, Brockley Cross Business Centre
96 Endwell Road

London, SE4 2PD
Telephone: (44) 020-7639-6967
http://www.childnet-int.org

This international website seeks to make the Internet a safe place for children and teens. Childnet International works around the world with many other organizations to help highlight and promote the many positive ways children and adolescents can use the Internet. The organization provides a wide range of strategic educational intervention and policy initiatives to protect younger generations.

Children's Partnership
Suite 206
1351 Third Street Promenade
Santa Monica, CA 90401
Telephone: 310-260-1220; Fax: 310-260-1921
http://www.childrenspartnership.org/

The Children's Partnership is a national nonprofit, nonpartisan organization that undertakes research, analysis, and advocacy to place the needs of U.S. children and youth, particularly the underserved, at the forefront of emerging policy debates. As part of its programming, the Children's Partnership provides an introduction to parenting in a world of computers and new forms of media. It provides some tools and rules for parents to use with their children at home, at school, and in the community.

Family Education Network
20 Park Plaza, Twelfth Floor
Boston, MA 02116
Telephone: 617-542-6500
http://familyeducation.com

The Family Education Network, launched in September 2000, is an extensive online network of learning and information resources, personalized to help parents, teachers, and students of all ages take control of their learning and make it part of their everyday lives. The Family Education Network as an extension of the international media company Pearson Learning Corporation, is funded by leading educational publishers and technology companies. Considerable information is available from the organization on the topics of Internet safety, chat rooms, and family rules for the use of the Internet.

Federal Bureau of Investigation
935 Pennsylvania Avenue NW, Room 11163
Washington, DC 20535
Telephone: 202-324-3666
http://www.fbi.gov/publications/pguide/pguidee.htm

The Federal Bureau of Investigation's online publication *A Parent's Guide to Internet Safety* is a resource guide that explains how advances in computer and telecommunication technology allow children and teenagers to reach out to new sources of knowledge and cultural experiences, but also how the Internet leaves them vulnerable to exploitation and harm by computer sex offenders. This source helps parents to understand the complexities of online child exploitation and where to go for advice and assistance.

GetNetWise
Internet Education Foundation
1634 Eye Street NW, Suite 1107
Washington, DC 20006
Telephone: 202-638-4370
http://www.getnetwise.org/

GetNetWise is a public service sponsored by various Internet industry corporations and public interest organizations to help ensure that families have safe, constructive, and educational or entertaining online experiences. The GetNetWise coalition wants Internet users to have full access to the resources they need to make informed decisions about their family's use of the Internet. GetNetWise is a project of the Internet Education Foundation.

Morality in Media
475 Riverside Drive, Suite 239
New York, NY 10115
Telephone: 212-870-3222; Fax: 212-870-2765
http://www.moralityinmedia.org/

Morality in Media is a national nonprofit interfaith organization established in 1962 to combat obscenity and to uphold decency standards in the media. It maintains the National Obscenity Law Center, a clearinghouse of legal materials on obscenity law, and conducts public information programs to educate and involve concerned citizens. Morality in Media seeks to promote the safe use of the Internet and prevent the sexual exploitation of children and teenagers.

National Center for Missing and Exploited Children
Charles B. Wang International Children's Building
699 Prince Street
Alexandria, VA 22314-3175
Telephone: 703-274-3900; Fax: 703-274-2200
http://www.missingkids.com/cybertip/index.html

The National Center for Missing and Exploited Children (NCMEC) is a private nonprofit organization that provides assistance to parents, children, law enforcement, schools, and the community in recovering missing children and in raising public awareness about ways to help prevent child abduction, molestation, and sexual exploitation. The NCMEC offers information designed to educate parents about the Internet as well as information on issues pertaining to children and teenagers using computers.

National Coalition for the Protection of Children and Families
800 Compton Road, Suite 9224
Cincinnati, OH 45231
Telephone: 513-521-6227
http://www.nationalcoalition.org/

The National Coalition for the Protection of Children and Families (NCPCF) is dedicated to helping people live lives that are free from the influences of pornography and the sexualized messages of the culture. Founded in 1983, this organization stresses how important it is for people to be educated on Internet safety issues and offers ways to deal with such problems as pornography and the sexual exploitation of children and adolescents.

Dating and Club Drugs

Addiction Resource Guide
P.O. Box 8612
Tarrytown, NY 10591
Telephone: 914-725-5151; Fax: 914-631-8077
http://www.addictionresourceguide.com/aboutthisguide.html

The Addiction Resource Guide is a website whose mission is to help professionals and consumers find resources for dealing with addictive problems, including club drugs. Website information includes residential treatment resources, self-help groups, and various publications.

American Society of Addiction Medicine
4601 North Park Avenue, Arcade Suite 101
Chevy Chase, MD 20815
Telephone: 301-656-3815; Fax: 301-656-3815
http://www.asam.org/Frames.htm

The American Society of Addiction Medicine is dedicated to educating physicians and improving the treatment of individuals
suffering from alcoholism or other addictions. It seeks to increase access to and improve the quality of addictions treatment; educate physicians, medical and osteopathic students,
and the public; and promote research and prevention. Considerable information on club drugs is available in the society's
archives.

Center for Alcohol and Addiction Studies
Box G-BH
Brown University
Providence, RI 02912
Telephone: 401-444-1800; Fax: 401-444-1850
http://www.caas.brown.edu/

The Center for Alcohol and Addiction Studies promotes the identification, prevention, and treatment of alcohol problems and
other drug use problems in society through research, education,
training, and policy advocacy. The center is located at Brown University's Butler Hospital campus in Providence, Rhode Island.

Center for Education and Drug Abuse Research
University of Pittsburgh
School of Pharmacy
711 Salk Hall
Pittsburgh, PA 15261
Telephone: 412-624-1060
http://cedar.pharmacy.pitt.edu/main.html

The mission of the Center for Education and Drug Abuse Research (CEDAR) is to identify and explain the causes and symptoms of substance abuse and substance use disorders. CEDAR is
funded by the National Institute on Drug Abuse. Adolescent
drug-taking behaviors are among the research areas explored at
the center.

Center for Treatment Research on Adolescent Drug Abuse
P.O. Box 019132
Miami, FL 33101
Telephone: 305-243-6434
http://www.miami.edu/UMH/CDA/UMH_Main/1,1770,7239
–1,00.html

The Center for Treatment Research on Adolescent Drug Abuse (CTRADA) began in 1991 as the first federally funded clinical research center focusing on adolescent drug abuse treatment. The center's overall goal is to conduct treatment research on adolescent drug abuse. CTRADA is funded by grants from the National Institute on Drug Abuse (NIDA) and the Center for Substance Abuse Treatment (CSAT). CTRADA is located on the University of Miami campus.

ClubDrugs.Org
National Institute on Drug Abuse
6001 Executive Boulevard, Room 5213
Bethesda, MD 20892-9561
Telephone: 301-443-1124
http://www.clubdrugs.org/

Sponsored by the National Institute on Drug Abuse (NIDA), this website provides scientific data gathered on the most prevalent club drugs. A comprehensive body of information explores how the use of club drugs can cause serious health problems and, in some cases, even death. Also included is information regarding the development of treatment and prevention strategies targeted to the populations that abuse club drugs.

Community Anti-Drug Coalitions of America (CADCA)
901 North Pitt Street, Suite 301
Alexandria, VA 22314
Telephone: 800-54-CADCA
http://www.cadca.org/

Community Anti-Drug Coalitions of America's mission is to build and strengthen the capacity of community coalitions to create safe, healthy, and drug-free communities. The organization provides technical assistance and training, public policy assistance, media strategies and marketing programs, conferences, and special events. Together, partners in each community organize and develop plans and programs to coordinate their antidrug efforts. The result is a comprehensive, community-wide approach to substance abuse and its related problems.

National Clearinghouse for Alcohol and Drug Information
11426 Rockville Pike, Suite 200
Rockville, MD 20849-6303
Telephone: 800-729-6686
http://www.health.org/

National Clearinghouse for Alcohol and Drug Information is the world's largest resource for current information and materials concerning alcohol and substance abuse prevention, intervention, and treatment. The National Clearinghouse for Alcohol and Drug Information (NCADI) is a service of the Center for Substance Abuse Prevention, which is under the Substance Abuse and Mental Health Services Administration (SAMHSA). Visitors to this website will find an abundance of information on club drugs.

National Council on Alcoholism and Drug Dependence
20 Exchange Place, Suite 2902
New York, NY 10005
Telephone: 212-269-7797; Fax: 212-269-7510
http://www.ncadd.org

Founded in 1944, the National Council on Alcoholism and Drug Dependence (NCADD) provides education, information, and assistance to the public. It advocates prevention, intervention, and treatment through offices in New York and Washington and through a nationwide network of affiliates.

Partnership for a Drug-Free America
405 Lexington Avenue, Suite 1601
New York, NY 10174
Telephone: 212-922-1560; Fax: 212-922-1570
http://www.drugfreeamerica.org/

The Partnership for a Drug-Free America seeks to help parents, adolescents, and children reject substance abuse. This website contains comprehensive and informative publications on all drugs, including such club drugs as Ecstasy. The organization provides parents with many details about Ecstasy, including its use, warning signs, short- term and long-term effects, and specific steps to help a teenager who is using the drug.

Date Rape

Alliance for Children and Families
Communications Department
11700 West Lake Park Drive
Milwaukee, WI 53224
Telephone: 414-359-1040 or 800-221-3726; Fax: 414-359-1074
http://www.alliance1.org

Formed in October 1998, the Alliance for Children and Families is an international membership association representing more than 350 private, nonprofit child- and family-serving organizations. Programs range from residential care to domestic abuse prevention and intervention. The alliance's mission is to strengthen members' capacity to serve and advocate for children, families, and communities.

Asian Task Force against Domestic Violence
P.O. Box 120108
Boston, MA 02112
Telephone: 617-338-2350; Fax: 617-338-2354
http://www.atask.org/

The Asian Task Force against Domestic Violence was founded in 1987 to address the need for multicultural and multilingual resources for Asian families facing domestic violence. The U.S. Department of Health and Human Services Office of Refugee Resettlement has identified domestic violence as one of the most serious problems facing Asian immigrant communities; the mission of the Asian Task Force against Domestic Violence is to eliminate family violence and to strengthen Asian families and communities. The Asian Task Force also provides information on date rape and stalking.

Family Violence and Sexual Assault Institute
7120 Herman Jared Drive
Forth Worth, TX 76180
Telephone: 817-569-8882; Fax: 817-485-0600
http://www.fvsai.org

The Family Violence and Sexual Assault Institute's mission is to improve the quality of life for individuals on an international level by sharing and disseminating information; improving networking among professionals; and assisting with program evaluation, consultation, and training that promotes violence-free living. The institute publishes the *Family Violence and Sexual Assault Bulletin,* the first publication focusing exclusively on family violence. Published quarterly and distributed internationally, it is a comprehensive periodical that addresses issues of family violence, sexual assault, and maltreatment of children and teens.

Family Violence Prevention Fund
383 Rhode Island Street, Suite 304
San Francisco, CA 94103-5133
Telephone: 415-252-8900
http://www.endabuse.org/

The Family Violence Prevention Fund works to prevent domestic violence and to help women and children whose lives are affected by abuse. The organization has piloted institutional change efforts, created public awareness campaigns, and developed public policy initiatives in the arenas of public health, child welfare, the law, public education, immigration, international settings, and the workplace. This website contains a wealth of information on date rape and stalking.

Men Stopping Rape, Inc.
306 North Brooks Street
Madison, WI 53715
Telephone: 608-257-4444
http://www.danenet.wicip.org/msr

Men Stopping Rape is an organization of men working in the Madison, Wisconsin community to promote education for men about sexual assault. Its membership consists of students at the University of Wisconsin, Madison campus as well as men working and living in the community. The membership embraces a wide range of ages, upbringings, orientations, and experiences. Members share a desire to live in a world free of violence against women and against men. Educational intervention includes publications, workshops, and seminars on all aspects of sexual assault.

National Coalition against Domestic Violence (NCADV)
P.O. Box 18749
Denver, CO 80218
Telephone: 303-839-1852; Fax: 303-831-925
http://www.ncadv.org/

The National Coalition against Domestic Violence (NCADV) is dedicated to the empowerment of battered women and their children and committed to the elimination of personal and societal violence in the lives of women and children. NCADV believes violence against women and children results from the use of force or threat to achieve and maintain control over others in intimate relationships, and from societal abuse of power in the forms of sexism, racism, homophobia, classism, anti-Semitism, able-body-ism, ageism, and other forms of discrimination. It is the mission of NCADV to work for the societal changes necessary to eliminate both personal and societal violence against all women and children.

National Council on Child Abuse and Family Violence
1155 Connecticut Avenue NW, Suite 400
Washington, DC 20036
Telephone: 202-429-6695 or 800-222-2000
http://www.nccafv.org/

The National Council on Child Abuse and Family Violence (NCCAFV) is a resource center on family violence prevention. NCCAFV offers a wide range of information on spouse/partner abuse, including date rape. NCCAFV provides public awareness and education materials, program and resource development consultation, and technical assistance and training in the United States and internationally.

National Sexual Violence Resource Center
123 North Enola Drive
Enola, PA 17025
Telephone: 877-739-3895 or 717-909-0710; Fax: 717-909-0714
http://www.nsvrc.org

Serving as a central clearinghouse for resources and research, the National Sexual Violence Resource Center (NSVRC) provides a source for information, help, and support. The NSVRC influences policy, practice, and research by providing greater interaction, investigation, and review and by promoting awareness within the anti-sexual violence movement. Working in concert with the University of Pennsylvania, the NSVRC provides review, analysis, and synthesis of the research being conducted in its field.

Office on Violence against Women
810 Seventh Street NW
Washington, DC 20531
Telephone: 202-307-6026; Fax: 202-307-3911
http://www.ojp.usdoj.gov/vawo/

Since its inception in 1995, the Office on Violence against Women has handled legal and policy issues regarding violence against women, provided national and international leadership, received international visitors interested in learning about the federal government's role in addressing violence against women, and responded to requests for information regarding violence against women. This website provides up-to-date information on interventions to stop violence against women; this information is of particular use to criminal justice practitioners, advocates, and social service professionals. The website also discusses research and promising practices regarding issues of domestic violence, date rape, stalking, batterer intervention programs, child custody and protection, sexual assault, and welfare reform.

Stalking Resource Center
National Center for Victims of Crime
2000 M Street NW, Suite 480
Washington, DC 20036
Telephone: 202-467-8700; Fax: 202-467-8701
http://www.ncvc.org/src/index.html

The Stalking Resource Center is a program sponsored by the National Center for Victims of Crime. The mission of the Stalking Resource Center is to raise national awareness of stalking and to encourage the development and implementation of multidisciplinary responses to stalking in local communities across the country. The center offers five specific program components: a peer-to-peer exchange program, training, an information clearinghouse, a practitioners' network, and a website.

Same-Sex Dating

Children of Lesbians and Gays Everywhere
3543 Eighteenth Street, Suite 1
San Francisco, CA 94110
Telephone: 415-861-5437; Fax: 415-255-8345
http://www.colage.org/

Children of Lesbians and Gays Everywhere works to make the world a better place for children of lesbian, gay, bisexual, and transgendered parents and families. The organization values a pluralistic definition of family and parent(s) encompassing a variety of kinship structures, including immediate families; extended families; partners; straight spouses; and family structures that are marginalized in American society such as single-parent families, multiracial families, international families, and families with disabilities.

Family Pride Coalition
P.O. Box 65327
Washington, DC 20035-5327
Telephone: 202-331-5015; Fax: 202-331-0080
http://www.familypride.org/

The mission of the Family Pride Coalition is to advance the well being of lesbian, gay, bisexual, and transgendered parents and their families through mutual support, community collaboration, and public understanding. The organization seeks to secure civil rights for families and other close relationships and to communicate its family values to the general public.

Gay and Lesbian Alliance against Defamation (GLAAD)
5455 Wilshire Boulevard, Suite 1500
Los Angeles, CA 90036
Telephone: 323-933-2240; Fax: 323-933-2241
http://www.glaad.org

The Gay and Lesbian Alliance against Defamation (GLAAD) is dedicated to promoting and ensuring fair, accurate, and inclusive representation of individuals and events in all media as a means of eliminating homophobia and discrimination based on gender identity and sexual orientation. GLAAD offers a wide range of programs, services, and publications.

Human Rights Campaign
919 Eighteenth Street NW, Suite 800
Washington, DC 20006
Telephone: 202-628-4160; Fax: 202-347-5323
http://www.hrcusa.org

The Human Rights Campaign is a bipartisan organization that works to advance equality based on sexual orientation and gender expression and identity, and to ensure that gay, lesbian, bisexual, and transgendered Americans can be open, honest, and safe at home, at work, and in the community. As the largest gay and lesbian organization in the United States, the Human Rights Campaign provides a national voice on gay and lesbian issues.

Institute for Gay and Lesbian Strategic Studies
P.O. Box 2603
Amherst, MA 01004-2603
Telephone: 413-577-0145
http://www.iglss.org/iglss/

The Institute for Gay and Lesbian Strategic Studies (IGLSS) promotes timely and relevant scholarship. Representing the lesbian, gay, bisexual, and transgender communities, IGLSS confronts important issues using credible methodology to ensure reliable answers. With a mix of scholarly study and data on important issues, IGLSS fulfills the research needs of the lesbian, gay, bisexual, and transgender communities and provides leadership within the movement through informed critical analysis.

National Gay and Lesbian Task Force
1325 Massachusetts Avenue NW, Suite 600
Washington, DC 20005
Telephone: 202-393-5177; Fax: 202-393-2241
http://www.ngltf.org/

The National Gay and Lesbian Task Force is a national progressive organization working for the civil rights of gay, lesbian, bisexual, and transgendered people. Among its programming efforts is a Policy Institute, which publishes original research, conducts analyses on existing data, engages in policy analysis, convenes roundtables of scholars and activists, and engages in public speaking and public education.

National Youth Advocacy Coalition
1638 R Street NW, Suite 300
Washington, DC 20009
Telephone: 202-319-7596; Fax: 202-319-7365
http://www.nyacyouth.org/

The National Youth Advocacy Coalition is a social justice organization that advocates for and with young people who are lesbian, gay, bisexual, transgendered, or questioning (LGBTQ), in an effort to end discrimination against these youths and to ensure their physical and emotional well being. The organization is committed to addressing the connections between race, gender, class, and sexual orientation and to bridging the gap that exists between adult LGBTQ civil rights organizations and the mainstream youth movement.

OutYouth
909 East 49 1/2 Street
Austin, TX 78751
Telephone: 512-419-1233; Fax: 512-419-1232
http://www.outyouth.org

OutYouth is a nonprofit organization providing services to gay, lesbian, bisexual, and transgendered youth ages 12 to 19 in Austin and the rest of central Texas. The organization offers peer support groups, counseling, educational programs, social activities, and community outreach to nurture adolescents' positive self-images and promote healthy, productive lives.

Parents, Families, and Friends of Lesbians and Gays
1726 M Street NW, Suite 400
Washington, DC 20036
Telephone: 202-467-8180; Fax: 202-467-8194
http://www.pflag.org/

Parents, Families, and Friends of Lesbians and Gays (PFLAG) is a national nonprofit organization with more than 80,000 members and supporters and more than 460 affiliates in the United States. This network is resourced and serviced by the PFLAG national office, located in Washington, D.C. PFLAG provides opportunity for dialogue about sexual orientation and gender identity, and it seeks to help create a society that is healthy and respectful of human diversity.

Project YES
5275 Sunset Drive
Miami, FL 33143
Telephone: 305-663-7195; Fax: 305-663-7197
http://www.projectyes.org/

Project YES is an educational organization whose mission is to prevent suicide and ensure the healthy development of gay, lesbian, bisexual, and transgendered youth by initiating dialogue, providing education, and creating support systems. Located in south Florida, Project YES conducts presentations and workshops both locally and nationally to give people ideas for making a difference. Project YES creates partnerships with corporations, hospitals, police departments, religious communities, schools, parent groups, and social service agencies.

Premarital Sex

Adolescent Reproductive Health
Program for Appropriate Technology in Health (PATH)
1455 Northwest Leary Way
Seattle, WA 98107-5136
Telephone: 206-285-3500; Fax: 206-285-6619
http://www.rho.org/html/adolescent.htm

Adolescent Reproductive Health provides up-to-date summaries of research findings, program experience, and clinical guidelines related to key reproductive health topics, as well as analyses of policy and program implications. The program works to improve the health and well being of young adults in developing countries through the creation and strengthening of effective reproductive health initiatives. An important objective of the organization is to help users link with quality online resources and collaborate with colleagues around the world.

Alan Guttmacher Institute (AGI)
120 Wall Street, Twenty-First Floor
New York, NY 10005
Telephone: 212-248-1111; Fax: 212-248-1951
http://www.agi-usa.org

The Alan Guttmacher Institute (AGI) is a nonprofit organization focused on sexual and reproductive health research, policy analysis, and public education. AGI publishes *Perspectives on Sexual and Reproductive Health, International Family Planning Perspectives, The Guttmacher Report on Public Policy,* and special reports on topics pertaining to sexual and reproductive health and rights. The institute's mission is to protect the reproductive choices of women and men in the United States and throughout the world. Its mission is to also support people's ability to obtain the information and services needed to achieve their full human rights, safeguard their health, and exercise their individual responsibilities in regard to sexual behavior and relationships, reproduction, and family formation.

Annie E. Casey Foundation
701 St. Paul Street
Baltimore, MD 21202
Telephone: 410-547-6600
http://www.aecf.org/

The Annie E. Casey Foundation (AECF) works to build better futures for disadvantaged children and their families in the United States. The primary mission of the foundation is to foster public policies, human service reforms, and community supports that more effectively meet the needs of todays vulnerable children and families. Focus areas include teenage pregnancy, parenthood, and reproduction.

Association of Reproductive Health Professionals
2401 Pennsylvania Avenue NW, Suite 350
Washington, DC 20037
Telephone: 202-466-3825; Fax: 202-466-3826
http://www.arhp.org/

The Association of Reproductive Health Professionals (ARHP) is a multidisciplinary association of professionals who provide reproductive health services or education, conduct reproductive health research, or influence reproductive health policy. ARHP educates healthcare professionals, policy makers, and the public. The organization fosters research and advocacy to improve reproductive health.

Center for Health and Gender Equity
6930 Carroll Avenue, Suite 910
Takoma Park, MD 20912

Telephone: 301-270-1182; Fax 301-270-2052
http://www.genderhealth.org/

This organization seeks to promote informed choices in the delivery of reproductive health technologies, including contraceptive methods and gender-sensitive approaches to the prevention of unwanted pregnancy, unsafe abortion, and sexually transmitted diseases. It also seeks to address gender-based violence and coercion as a key factor in high rates of reproductive morbidity and mortality and as a violation of women's fundamental human rights, and to promote the development of equitable health systems through health sector reforms that are responsive to reproductive and sexual rights concerns.

ETR Associates
4 Carbonero Way
Scotts Valley, CA 95066-4200
Telephone: 800-321-4407; Fax: 1-800-435-8433
http://www.etr.org

ETR (Education, Training, and Research) Associates seeks to encourage young people and adults to adopt positive attitudes and behaviors that contribute to optimal sexual health and well being. ETR considers the development of positive family and peer relationships essential to well being. The organization strives to make available sexuality education that results in fulfilling and responsible interpersonal, sexual, and reproductive behavior. ETR Associates offers products and services in five primary areas: resources development, publishing and distribution, research and evaluation, program development and training, and clearinghouse services.

Go Ask Alice!
Lerner Hall
2920 Broadway, Seventh Floor
MC 2608
New York, NY 10027
Telephone: 212-854-5453
http://www.goaskalice.columbia.edu

Go Ask Alice! is a website offering comprehensive dating and sexuality information, including issues related to premarital sexual relationships. The mission of Go Ask Alice! is to increase access to, and use of, health information by providing factual, in-depth, straightforward, and nonjudgmental information to assist readers' decision making about their physical, sexual, emotional, and spiritual health. The website is maintained by Columbia University health educators.

National Campaign to Prevent Teen Pregnancy
1776 Massachusetts Avenue NW, Suite 200
Washington, DC 20036
Telephone: 202-478-8500; Fax: 202-478-8588
http://www.teenpregnancy.org/

The National Campaign to Prevent Teen Pregnancy is a nonprofit, nonpartisan initiative supported almost entirely by private donations. Its mission is to improve the well being of children, youth, and families by reducing teen pregnancy. To accomplish this, the campaign provides a national presence and leadership to raise awareness of the issue and to attract new voices and resources to the cause. It also provides concrete assistance to those already working in the field. The campaign also tries to ease the many disagreements that have plagued both national and local efforts to address this problem.

National Family Planning and Reproductive Health Association (NFPRHA)
1627 K Street NW, Twelfth Floor
Washington, DC 20006
Telephone: 202-293-3114
http://www.nfprha.org/

The National Family Planning and Reproductive Health Association (NFPRHA) is a national nonprofit organization that works to ensure access to voluntary family planning and reproductive healthcare services and to support reproductive freedom. NFPRHA represents most of the domestic family planning field, including clinicians, administrators, researchers, educators, advocates, and consumers. NFPRHA members provide reproductive healthcare to nearly 5 million low-income women each year at more than 4,200 clinics nationwide.

Network for Family Life Education
Rutgers University
100 Joyce Kilmer Avenue

Piscataway, NJ 08854
Telephone: 732-445-7929; Fax: 732-445-4154
http://www.sxetc.org/whoweare/genWhoNFLE.asp

The Network for Family Life Education, a creation of Rutgers University, was founded in 1981. Its mission is to help children and youth become sexually healthy people and avoid pregnancy and disease during their teenage years. The network carries out this mission by providing educational resources, training, and technical assistance and by advocating for comprehensive sexuality education in schools and communities.

Planned Parenthood Federation of America
810 Seventh Avenue
New York, NY 10019
Telephone: 212-541-7800; Fax: 212-541-7800
http://www.plannedparenthood.org/

Planned Parenthood provides comprehensive reproductive and healthcare services in settings that preserve and protect the essential privacy and rights of each individual. The organization advocates public policies that guarantee these rights and provides educational programs that enhance understanding of individual and societal implications of human sexuality. Planned Parenthood also promotes research and the advancement of technology in reproductive healthcare.

Teenwire.com
Planned Parenthood Federation of America
810 Seventh Avenue
New York, NY 10019
Telephone: 212-541-7800; Fax: 212-541-7800
http://www.teenwire.com/

Teenwire.com is a website for adolescents offering information about all aspects of sexual health and well being. This website provides facts about sex so that teenagers can use this information to make their own responsible choices. Clear, honest, and nonjudgmental information about sexuality is provided with the hope that adolescents will use this knowledge to reduce their risk of unintended pregnancy and sexually transmitted diseases.

Birth Control

Center for Development and Population Activities
1400 Sixteenth Street NW, Suite 100
Washington, DC 20036
Telephone: 202-667-1142; Fax: 202-332-4496
http://www.cedpa.org/

The Center for Development and Population Activities (CEDPA) was founded in 1975 and has provided services to millions of women through partnerships with 138 organizations in 40 countries. The center helps ensure access to high-quality reproductive health services and voluntary family planning. The center strengthens community organizations that provide those choices and other vital support. Leaders of those groups form a global network and join together with CEDPA at national and global levels.

Contraceptive Research and Development Program (CONRAD)
Eastern Virginia Medical School
1611 North Kent Street, Suite 806
Arlington, VA 22209
Telephone: 703-524-4744; Fax: 703-524-4770
http://www.conrad.org/

The Contraceptive Research and Development Program (CONRAD) is dedicated to developing better, safer, and more acceptable methods of contraception that are especially suitable for use in developing countries. The ultimate goal of CONRAD's research is to improve reproductive health by expanding the contraceptive choices of women and men and by helping to prevent the transmission of HIV/AIDS and other sexually transmitted diseases. CONRAD was established in 1986 through a cooperative agreement between Eastern Virginia Medical School in Norfolk and the U.S. Agency for International Development. The organization works in collaboration with investigators at universities, research institutes, and private companies worldwide.

EngenderHealth
440 Ninth Avenue, Third Floor
New York, NY 10001
Telephone: 212-561-8000; Fax: 212-561-8067
http://www.engenderhealth.org/index.html

EngenderHealth works worldwide to make reproductive health services safe, available, and sustainable. The organization believes that individuals have the right to make informed decisions about their reproductive health and to receive care that meets their needs. EngenderHealth works in partnership with governments, institutions, and health care professionals to make this right a reality. The organization offers programming in maternal and child health, contraception, and gender issues.

Family Care International
588 Broadway, Suite 503
New York, NY 10012
Telephone: 212-941-5300; Fax: 212-941-5563
http://www.familycareintl.org/about/index.html

Family Care International is dedicated to improving women's sexual and reproductive health and rights in developing countries, with a special emphasis on making pregnancy and childbirth safer. A major program component is seeking to make comprehensive sexual and reproductive health information, education, support, and services available to adolescents around the world.

Family Health International
P.O. Box 13950
Research Triangle Park, NC 27709
Telephone: 919-544-7040; Fax: 919-544-7261
http://www.fhi.org/splash.htm

Family Health International (FHI) works to improve reproductive and family health around the world through biomedical and social science research, innovative health service delivery interventions, training, and information programs. FHI works in partnership with universities, ministries of health, nongovernmental organizations, and faith-based organizations, conducting ongoing projects in the United States and more than sixty developing countries. FHI works to improve the safety, efficacy, and acceptability of family planning methods and the quality and accessibility of reproductive health services.

Global Reproductive Health Forum
Harvard School of Public Health
Department of Population and International Health

665 Huntington Avenue
Boston, MA 02115
Telephone: 617-432-4619
http://www.hsph.harvard.edu/grhf/

The Global Reproductive Health Forum (GRHF) is an Internet networking project that aims to encourage critical discussions about reproductive health and gender on the Internet. GRHF provides interactive electronic forums and global discussions, distributes reproductive health and rights materials from a variety of perspectives through its clearinghouse, and maintains an extensive, up-to-date research library. Its goal is to reach out to, involve, and meet the needs of underserved groups, the reproductive health community, academics, and anyone dedicated to women's rights and gender issues.

Institute for Reproductive Health
Georgetown University
4301 Connecticut Avenue NW, Suite 310
Washington, DC 20008
Telephone: 202-687-1392; Fax: 202-537-7450
http://www.irh.org/

The Institute for Reproductive Health is dedicated to helping women and men make informed choices about family planning and providing them with simple and effective natural options. As part of Georgetown University's School of Medicine, the institute conducts research to develop natural methods of family planning and test them in service delivery settings. The institute's goal is to make natural methods easier to use and more widely available.

JHPIEGO Corporation
1615 Thames Street, Suite 200
Baltimore, MD 21231
Telephone: 410-537-1800; Fax: 410-537-1474
http://www.irh.org/index.html

Through advocacy, education, and performance improvement, JHPIEGO helps host-country policy makers, educators, and trainers increase access and reduce barriers to quality health services, especially family planning and maternal and neonatal care, for all members of their nations. JHPIEGO encourages innovative and practical solutions to meet identified needs in low-resource settings throughout Africa, Asia, Latin America, and the Caribbean.

Office of Population Research
Princeton University, Wallace Hall
Princeton, NJ 08544
Telephone: 609-258-4870; Fax: 609-258-1039
http://www.opr.princeton.edu/

The Office of Population Research (OPR) at Princeton University is a leading demographic research and training center. OPR makes contributions in formal demography and the study of fertility change, as well as trends in contraception. In recent years, there has been increasing research activity in the areas of health and well being, social demography, and migration and urbanization.

Population Action International
1300 Nineteenth Street NW, Second Floor
Washington, DC 20036
Telephone: 202-557-3400; Fax: 202-728-4177
http://www.populationaction.org/

Population Action International (PAI) fosters the development of United States and international policy on urgent population and reproductive health issues through an integrated program of research, advocacy, and communications. PAI seeks to make clear the linkages between population, reproductive health, the environment, and development. PAI shares its findings through the dissemination of strategic, action-oriented publications; participation in and sponsoring of conferences, meetings and seminars; and other efforts to educate and inform policy makers and the general public as well as colleagues in the health, environment, development, and related fields around the world.

Population Institute
107 Second Street NE
Washington, DC 20002
Telephone: 202-544-3300; Fax: 202-544-0068
http://www.populationinstitute.org/

The Population Institute is an international, educational, non-profit organization that seeks to reduce excessive population growth. The organization strives to achieve a world population in balance with a healthy global environment and resource base. Established in 1969, the institute offers a wide range of information, including material related to fertility, contraception, and reproduction policies around the globe.

Population Reference Bureau
1875 Connecticut Avenue NW, Suite 520
Washington, DC 20009-5728
Telephone: 1-800-877-9881; Fax: 202-328-3937
http://www.prb.org/

The Population Reference Bureau (PRB) provides timely and objective information on U.S. and international population trends and their implications, including contraception and family planning. PRB informs policy makers, educators, the media, and concerned citizens working in the public interest around the world through a broad range of activities, including publications, information services, seminars and workshops, and technical support.

Teenage Pregnancy

Adolescence Directory On-Line
Center for Adolescent Studies
School of Education, Indiana University
Bloomington, IN 47405
Telephone: 812-856-8113
http://www.education.indiana.edu/cas/adol/adol.html

Adolescence Directory on Line (ADOL) is an electronic guide to information on adolescent issues. It is a service of the Center for Adolescent Studies at Indiana University. Educators, counselors, parents, researchers, health practitioners, and teens can use ADOL to find Web resources on the topics of adolescent sexuality, pregnancy, and sexually transmitted diseases.

Best Friends Foundation
4455 Connecticut Avenue NW, Suite 310
Washington, DC 20008
Telephone: 202-237-8156
http://www.bestfriendsfoundation.org/

Best Friends is a youth development program with a character-building curriculum for girls in grades 5–12 with messages of abstinence from sex, drugs, and alcohol. Best Friends is an in-school program conducted during the school day by educators who serve as instructors and mentors. The program provides activities that help adolescent girls develop the skills necessary to avoid risk behaviors and become socially competent individuals.

Campaign for Our Children
120 West Fayette Street, Suite 1200
Baltimore, MD 21201
Telephone: 410-576-9015
http://www.cfoc.org/

Campaign for Our Children (CFOC) is a national nonprofit organization that creates educational media campaigns designed to promote adolescent preventive health issues. CFOC was formed in 1987 and directs much of its attention to implementing a comprehensive campaign to reduce teen pregnancy in Maryland. CFOC works hand in hand with the state to accomplish its mission with mass media and hands-on educational activities for classrooms and communities.

Center on Adolescent Sexuality, Pregnancy, and Parenting
162B Stanley Hall, University of Missouri
Columbia, MO 65211
Telephone: 573-882-3243; Fax: 573-884-4878
http://www.outreach.missouri.edu/hdfs/caspp.htm

The Center on Adolescent Sexuality, Pregnancy, and Parenting has a multidisciplinary team of professionals who provide educational programs and conduct applied research to better understand how to prevent and ameliorate the negative effects of high-risk sexual behaviors and early childbearing. This program is supported by the University of Missouri Outreach and Extension Outreach Development Fund.

Girls Incorporated
120 Wall Street
New York, NY 10005-3902
Telephone: 800-374-4475
http://www.girlsinc.org/

Girls Incorporated is a national nonprofit youth organization dedicated to inspiring all girls to be strong, smart, and bold. Girls Incorporated provides educational programs to American girls, particularly those in high-risk, underserved areas. Its programs, including pregnancy and drug abuse prevention, helps girls confront subtle societal messages about their value and potential, and prepare them to lead successful, independent, and fulfilling lives.

**Maltreatment and Adolescent Pregnancy
and Parenting Program**
314 Gentry Hall
University of Missouri Outreach and Extension
Columbia, MO 65211
Telephone: 573-882-6802; Fax: 573-884-4878
http://www.outreach.missouri.edu/hdfs/mappp/index.htm

The Maltreatment and Adolescent Pregnancy and Parenting Program (MAPPP) builds community awareness about the prevalence of violence in the lives of young women. MAPPP focuses its attention on three areas: the relationship between child maltreatment and later adolescent pregnancy, the factors associated with maltreatment of pregnant adolescents, and the likelihood that children of adolescent mothers will experience maltreatment.

National Network for Youth
1319 F Street NW, Fourth Floor
Washington, DC 20004-1106
Telephone: 202-783-7949; Fax: 202-783-7955
http://www.nn4youth.org/my/shared/home.jsp

The National Network for Youth is dedicated to ensuring that young people can be safe and lead healthy and productive lives, especially those who, because of life circumstance, disadvantage, past abuse, or community prejudice, have less opportunity to become contributing members of their communities. The network believes in healthy, positive alternatives for all youth and believes that young people can and will make informed choices concerning their own health and futures, including their sexual lives.

**National Organization on Adolescent Pregnancy,
Parenting, and Prevention**
2401 Pennsylvania Avenue NW, Suite 350
Washington, DC 20037
Telephone: 202-293-8370; Fax: 202-293-8805
http://www.noappp.org/

The National Organization on Adolescent Pregnancy, Parenting, and Prevention (NOAPPP) provides general leadership, education, training, information, advocacy, resources, and support to individuals and organizations in the field of adolescent pregnancy, parenting, and prevention. Inherent in its mission is the belief that effective adolescent pregnancy prevention, pregnancy programs, and parenting programs are comprehensive, utilize research-based strategies, demonstrate an understanding and respect for the rights and capabilities of adolescents, and include a range of stake holders in the decision making, implementation, and evaluation processes.

National Teen Pregnancy Prevention Research Center
University Gateway Building
Division of General Pediatrics and Adolescent Health
200 Oak Street SE, Suite 260
Minneapolis, MN 55455-2002
Telephone: 612-625-1674; Fax: 612-626-2134
http://www.prc.umn.edu

The National Teen Pregnancy Prevention Research Center is a collaborative effort by the schools of Medicine, Public Health, and Nursing and the Carlson School of Management at the University of Minnesota to provide interdisciplinary training to pregnancy prevention researchers and practitioners. The center is funded by the Centers for Disease Control and Prevention. The center partners with local, state, and national pregnancy prevention and youth-serving organizations to facilitate extensive dissemination of research findings on best programs and practices related to teenage pregnancy prevention.

Not Me, Not Now
40 Wildbrier Road
Henrietta, NY 14614
Telephone: 585-334-0890; Fax: 585-334-0855
http://www.notmenotnow.org/

Not Me, Not Now is a program that focuses on helping adolescents make important personal decisions, with a particular emphasis placed on whether to become sexually active. Not Me, Not Now helps adolescents become more aware of the consequences of teenage pregnancy and how to resist peer and other social pressure. An important program component is aimed at parents and how they can develop better communication skills to talk with their teens about sex and other personal issues.

Sexually Transmitted Diseases

AIDSinfo
P.O. Box 6303
Rockville, MD 20849-6303
Telephone: 800-448-0440; Fax: 301-519-6616
http://www.aidsinfo.nih.gov/

AIDSinfo is a U.S. Department of Health and Human Services (DHHS) project providing information on HIV/AIDS clinical trials and treatment. It is the result of merging two previous DHHS projects: the AIDS Clinical Trials Information Service (ACTIS) and the HIV/AIDS Treatment Information Service (ATIS). AIDSinfo is a central resource for current information on federally and privately funded clinical trials for AIDS patients and others infected with HIV.

AIDS Health Project
1855 Folsom Street, Suite 670
San Francisco, CA 94103
Telephone: 415-476-3902
http://www.ucsf-ahp.org/

The AIDS Health Project is affiliated with the University of California, San Francisco and San Francisco General Hospital. The AIDS Health Project provides direct mental health services to people with HIV; friends, family members, and partners of people with HIV; and caregivers. To share its experience and magnify the effects of its expertise, the AIDS Health Project also has developed an extensive education program for mental health providers.

American Foundation for AIDS Research (amfAR)
120 Wall Street, Thirteenth Floor
New York, NY 10005-3902
Telephone: 212-806-1600; Fax: 212-806-1601
http://www.amfar.org

The American Foundation for AIDS Research (amfAR) is a nonprofit organization dedicated to the support of HIV/AIDS research, AIDS prevention, treatment education, and the advocacy of sound AIDS-related public policy. The organization has active programs in basic research, clinical research and information, public and professional education, public policy, prevention science, and global initiatives. Funded by voluntary contributions from individuals, foundations, and corporations, amfAR has invested nearly $190 million in support of its mission since 1985 and has funded grants to more than 1,900 research teams worldwide.

American Social Health Association
P.O. Box 13827
Research Triangle Park, NC 27709
Telephone: 919-361-8400; Fax: 919-361-8425
http://www.ashastd.org/

The American Social Health Association (ASHA) develops and delivers accurate, medically reliable information about STDs. ASHA provides educational pamphlets and books to public and college health clinics to distribute to their clients and students. ASHA also helps community-based organizations communicate about risk, transmission, prevention, testing, and treatment. The ASHA offers facts, support, and resources to answer questions, find referrals, join help groups, and get access to in-depth information about sexually transmitted diseases.

CDC National Prevention Information Network
P.O. Box 6003
Rockville, MD 20849-6003
Telephone: 800-458-5231; Fax: 1-888-282-7681
http://www.cdcnpin.org/

The CDC National Prevention Information Network (NPIN) is the U.S. reference, referral, and distribution service for information on HIV/AIDS and other sexually transmitted diseases. NPIN produces, collects, catalogs, processes, stocks, and disseminates materials and information and offers a number of specialized services including searchable databases, reference and referral services, the website, resource centers, a free fax service, and a resource service for business and labor groups. All NPIN services are designed to facilitate sharing of information and resources on education and prevention services, published materials, research findings, and trends among users.

Center for AIDS Prevention Studies
University of California, San Francisco
74 New Montgomery, Suite 600
San Francisco, CA 94105
Telephone: 415-597-9100; Fax: 415-597-9213
http://www.caps.ucsf.edu

The mission of the Center for AIDS Prevention Studies (CAPS) is to conduct theory-based research that will have maximum impact on the theory, practice, and policy of AIDS prevention. CAPS stimulates new research projects to keep pace with the epidemic, provide necessary services to existing research projects and to the scientists at the center, and provide a platform for scientific interactions to advance and enhance multidisciplinary research in AIDS prevention.

Center for Health Services
Management Sciences for Health
165 Allandale Road
Boston, MA 02130
Telephone: 617-524-7799; Fax: 617-524-2825
http://www.msh.org/what_MSH_does/chs/index.html

The Center for Health Services works to improve the management and delivery of child survival, maternal health, and reproductive health services. Topics of interest of this organization include safer sex and the prevention of sexually transmitted diseases, including the global epidemic of HIV/AIDS. The Center for Health Services collaborates with and supports the efforts of government agencies at all levels, nongovernmental organizations, and the private sector to foster innovative approaches.

Division of Sexually Transmitted Diseases
Centers for Disease Control and Prevention
1600 Clifton Road
Atlanta, GA 30333
Telephone: 404-639-3311
http://www.cdc.gov/nchstp/dstd/dstdp.html

The Division of STD Prevention at the Centers for Disease Control and Prevention provides national leadership through research, policy development, and support of effective services to prevent sexually transmitted diseases (including HIV infection) and their complications, such as enhanced HIV transmission, infertility, adverse outcomes of pregnancy, and reproductive tract cancer. The Division of Sexually Transmitted Diseases assists health departments, healthcare providers, and nongovernmental organizations and collaborates with other governmental entities through the development, syntheses, translation, and dissemination of timely, science-based information; the development of national goals and science-based policy; and the development and support of science-based programs that meet the needs of communities.

Medical Institute for Sexual Health
P.O. Box 162306
Austin, TX 78716-2306
Telephone: 512-328-6268; Fax: 512-328-6269
http://www.medinstitute.org/

The Medical Institute for Sexual Health identifies, evaluates, and communicates credible scientific data to promote healthy sexual decisions and behavior in order to improve the welfare of individuals and society. A nonprofit medical organization founded in 1992, the Medical Institute confronts the worldwide epidemics of unwanted pregnancy and sexually transmitted disease with incisive healthcare data.

Mothers' Voices
165 West Forty-Sixth Street, Suite 701
New York, NY 10036
Telephone: 212-730-2777; Fax: 212-730-4378
http://www.mvoices.org/

Mothers' Voices is a national nonprofit organization that believes every child deserves a full and healthy life, free of HIV/AIDS. The organization seeks to mobilize parents and other concerned individuals to be educators and advocates dedicated to the prevention of HIV infection in all children. As such, Mothers' Voices promotes public policies that advance efforts for AIDS education, prevention, research, treatment, and, ultimately, a cure.

TeenAIDS
P.O. Box 146727
Boston, MA 02114
Telephone: 978-665-9383

http://4www.teenAIDS.org

TeenAIDS is a nonprofit organization dedicated to educating teens around the world about the prevention of HIV/AIDS. Maintained by PeerCorps with technological support from Harvard University and MIT, TeenAIDS seeks to empower teens to protect themselves and their friends from HIV infection. The organization uses a combination of personal contact and the Internet to spread its message locally and globally. The TeenAIDS website can be viewed in English, Spanish, French, Portuguese, Chinese, German, Italian, and Vietnamese.

Living Together

Alternatives to Marriage Project
P.O. Box 991010
Boston, MA 02199
Telephone 781-793-0296; Fax 781-394-6625
http://www.unmarried.org

The Alternatives to Marriage Project (AtMP) advocates for equality and fairness for unmarried people, including people who choose not to marry, who cannot marry, or who live together before marriage. The project provides support and information, fights discrimination on the basis of marital status, and educates the public and policy makers about relevant social and economic issues. The organization believes that marriage is only one of many acceptable family forms and that society should recognize and support healthy relationships in all their diversity.

Coalition for Marriage, Family, and Couples Education
5310 Belt Road NW
Washington, DC 20015-1961
Telephone: 202-362-3332; Fax: 202-362-0973
http://www.smartmarriages.com/

The Coalition for Marriage, Family, and Couples Education (CMFCE) is an independent, nonpartisan, nondenominational, and nonsectarian organization. It seeks to enhance and strengthen couple and family relationships through education and information. The coalition offers a number of publications and programming endeavors related to all variations of marriage and family life.

Couple Communication
Interpersonal Communication Programs, Inc. (ICP)
30772 Southview Drive, Suite 200
Evergreen, CO 80439
Telephone: 303-674-2051; Fax: 303-674-4283
http://www.couplecommunication.com/

Couple Communication began at the University of Minnesota Family Study Center in 1972 and bases its program concepts, skills, and processes on communication and systems theory. The program provides exercises, guidance, and assorted materials to help couples communicate skillfully, resolve conflicts collaboratively, and build satisfying relationships with family, friends, and people at work. To date, more than 70 published studies have demonstrated the practicality and positive effects of the concepts and skills of the program.

Family and Home Network
9493C Silver King Court
Fairfax, VA 22031
Telephone: 703-352-1072; Fax: 703-352-1076
http://www.familyandhome.org/

Family and Home Network is a national nonprofit organization founded in 1984. Family and Home Network publishes books and informative collections of articles on a range of family life topics. In addition to its own publishing ventures, the organization seeks to educate the reading public, members of the media, and policy makers about families from all walks of life.

Family Diversity Projects
P.O. Box 1246
Amherst, MA 01004-1246
Telephone: 413-256-0502; Fax: 413-253-3977
http://www.familydiv.org/

Family Diversity Projects seeks to promote a multicultural understanding of intimate relationships. Through books and artwork, Family Diversity Projects celebrates families of every kind, including adoptive families, foster families, multiracial families, physically challenged families, lesbian- and gay-parented families, interfaith families, multigenerational families and others.

Family Information Services
12565 Jefferson Street NE, Suite 102
Minneapolis, MN 55434
Telephone: 763-755-6233; Fax: 763-755-7355
http://www.familyinfoserv.com/index.html

Family Information Services is an independent organization dedicated exclusively to the continuing education of parent and family life educators. The organization offers ideas and strategies for working with parents, children, youth, couples, and/or families. It offers a variety of informational resources, newsletters, and continuing education opportunities.

Institute for 21st Century Relationships
2419 Little Current Drive, Suite 1933
Herndon, VA 20171-4612
Telephone: 703-561-8136; Fax: 703-561-8336
http://www.lovethatworks.org/

The Institute for 21st Century Relationships works to help people fulfill their potential for relating and to support people's freedom to discover and practice the intimate relationship structure that best meets their needs. The institute utilizes research and educational support to create a climate in which all forms of ethical, consensual, and fulfilling relationship styles are broadly understood and are equally respected and honored as legitimate life choices.

LifePartners
6770 Eagle Ridge Road
Penngrove, CA 94951-9728
Telephone: 707-792-6700
http://www.lifepartners.com/

LifePartners was founded in 1989 with the intent of offering relationship skill building through workshops, seminars, and assorted publications. Readers will find a variety of relationship resources, including those aimed at communication skills, conflict resolution, and child rearing issues.

National Council on Family Relations
3989 Central Avenue NE, Suite 550
Minneapolis, MN 55421

Telephone: 763-781-9331; Fax: 763-781-9348
http://www.ncfr.com/

The National Council on Family Relations (NCFR) provides a forum for family researchers, educators, and practitioners to share in the development and dissemination of knowledge about families and family relationships. It also establishes professional standards, and works to promote family well being. The organization's two publications, the *Journal of Marriage and Family* and *Family Relations*, regularly feature articles on many different aspects of cohabitation, including adjustment issues.

PAIRS Foundation
1056 Creekford Drive
Weston, FL 33326
Telephone: 888-724-7748; Fax: 954-389-9596
http://www.pairsfoundation.com/contact.html

The PAIRS (Practical Application of Intimate Relationship Skills) program provides a comprehensive psychoeducational approach designed to enhance self-knowledge and to develop the ability of participants to sustain rewarding intimate relationships. The PAIRS approach integrates a wide range of theories and methods such as psychology, education, and psychotherapy and presents them in an educational format. The organization also offers a variety of publications on relationship skill building.

Teenage Marriages

Administration for Children and Families
U.S. Department of Health and Human Services
200 Independence Avenue SW
Washington, D.C. 20201
Telephone: 202-619-0257 or 877-696-6775
http://www.acf.dhhs.gov/index.html

The Administration for Children and Families (ACF) is a federal agency funding state, local, and tribal organizations to provide family assistance (welfare), child support, child care, Head Start, child welfare, and other programs relating to children and families. The website features such adolescent research areas as pregnancy, marriage, and sexually transmitted diseases.

Alliance for Young Families
105 Chauncy Street, Eighth Floor
Boston, MA 02111
Telephone: 617-482-912; Fax: 617-482-9129
http://www.youngfamilies.org

The mission of the Alliance for Young Families is to provide statewide leadership to prevent adolescent pregnancy and to promote quality services for pregnant and parenting teens and their children through policy analysis, education, research, and advocacy. The alliance is a nonprofit coalition of approximately 100 health and human service agencies.

American Association for Marriage and Family Therapy
112 South Alfred Street
Alexandria, VA 22314-3061
Telephone: 703-838-9808; Fax: 703-838-9805
http://www.aamft.org

The American Association for Marriage and Family Therapy (AAMFT) is the professional association for practitioners in the field of marriage and family therapy. Its major publication, the *Journal of Marital and Family Therapy*, often focuses on adjustments to marriage, including those inherent in adolescent relationships. The AAMFT represents the professional interests of more than 23,000 marriage and family therapists throughout the United States, Canada, and abroad.

Center for the Improvement of Child Caring (CICC)
11331 Ventura Boulevard, Suite 103
Studio City, CA 91604-3147
Telephone: 818-980-0903; Fax: 818-753-1054
http://www.ciccparenting.org/

The Center for the Improvement of Child Caring (CICC) is a parenting and parenting education organization established in 1974. It is a private, nonprofit community service, training, and research corporation and a major supporter and participant in a nationwide movement to improve the overall quality of child rearing and child caring in the United States.

Children's Rights Council
6200 Editors Park Drive, Suite 103

Hyattsville, MD 20782
Telephone: 301-559-3120; Fax: 301-559-3124
http://www.info4parents.com/index.html

Formed in 1985, the Children's Rights Council (CRC) is a national nonprofit organization based in Washington, D.C., that works to ensure that children have meaningful and continuing contact with their parent(s) and with their extended families, regardless of the parents' marital status. The organization publishes a quarterly newsletter; testifies on behalf of the organization's positions before the U.S. Congress; communicates with the national media; provides published materials including books, briefs, and cassettes consistent with its purpose; meets with policy makers throughout the country; and generally educates people about prevalent practices in U.S. courts and departments of human services and how these practices can affect children's family situations.

Family and Youth Services Bureau
U.S. Department of Health and Human Services
P.O. Box 1882
Washington, DC 20013
Telephone: 202-205-8102; Fax: 202-260-9333
http://www.ojjdp.ncjrs.org/pubs/fedresources/ag–04.html

The Family and Youth Services Bureau (FYSB) is an agency within the Administration for Children and Families. FYSB provides national leadership on youth-related issues and helps individuals and organizations to provide comprehensive services for youths in at-risk situations as well as for their families. The primary goals of FYSB programs are to provide positive alternatives for youth, ensure their safety, and maximize their potential to take advantage of available opportunities. FYSB programs and services support locally based youth services.

FamilyCares
Points of Light Foundation
1400 I Street NW, Suite 800
Washington, DC 20005-2208
Telephone: 202-729-8000; Fax: 202-729-8100
http://www.pointsoflight.org/

FamilyCares is part of the Points of Light Foundation, a national, nonpartisan, nonprofit organization that promotes volunteerism.

The FamilyCares program helps to promote compassion through hands-on family projects that help others in need. Based in Washington, D.C., the FamilyCares program advocates community service through a partnership with the Volunteer Center National Network.

Family Support America
20 North Wacker Drive, Suite 1100
Chicago, IL 60606
Telephone: 312-338-0900; Fax: 312-338-1522
http://www.familysupportamerica.org/

Family Support America works to strengthen and support families and places the principles of family support practice at the heart of every setting in which children and families are present. Particular attention is given to the education of young parents and to the health and well being of their children.

National Center on Fathers and Families
University of Pennsylvania
3440 Market Street, Suite 450
Philadelphia, PA 19104-3325
Telephone: 215-573-5500
http://www.ncoff.gse.upenn.edu/

The National Center on Fathers and Families (NCOFF) was established in 1994 at the Graduate School of Education, University of Pennsylvania, with core support from the Annie E. Casey Foundation. An interdisciplinary policy research center, NCOFF is dedicated to research and practice that expands the knowledge base on father involvement and family development and that informs policy designed to improve the well being of children.

National Clearinghouse on Families and Youth
P.O. Box 13505
Silver Spring, MD 20911-3505
Telephone: 301-608-8098; Fax: 301-608-8721
http://www.ncfy.com/index.htm

The Family and Youth Services Bureau (FYSB) established the National Clearinghouse on Families and Youth (NCFY) to assist individuals seeking to support young people and their families. The National Clearinghouse on Families and Youth is a comprehensive resource center and provides information on a wide range of family issues, including young people's marriages.

National Fatherhood Initiative
101 Lake Forest Boulevard, Suite 360
Gaithersburg, MD 20877
Telephone: 301-948-0599; Fax: 301-948-4325
http://www.fatherhood.org/

The National Fatherhood Initiative (NFI) was founded in 1994 to confront the problem of father absence. NFI's mission is to increase the proportion of children growing up with involved, responsible, and committed fathers. NFI works to accomplish this mission by educating people through public awareness campaigns, research, and other resources; equipping and developing leaders of fatherhood initiatives through curricula, training, and technical assistance; and engaging every sector of society through strategic alliances and partnerships.

Dating and Sexuality Education

American Association of Sexuality Educators,
Counselors, and Therapists
P.O. Box 5488
Richmond, VA 23220-0488
Telephone: 703-524-3287
http://www.aasect.org

The American Association of Sex Educators, Counselors, and Therapists (AASECT) is a not-for-profit interdisciplinary professional organization. In addition to sexuality educators and sex therapists, AASECT members include physicians, nurses, social workers, psychologists, allied health professionals, clergy members, lawyers, sociologists, marriage and family counselors and therapists, family planning specialists and researchers, and students in relevant professional disciplines. These individuals share an interest in promoting understanding of human sexuality and healthy sexual behavior.

Girls Incorporated
120 Wall Street
New York, NY 10005

Telephone: 212-509-2000
http://www.girlsinc.org/

Girls Incorporated develops research-based informal education programs that encourage girls to master physical, intellectual, and emotional challenges. Major programs address math and science education, pregnancy and drug abuse prevention, media literacy, economic literacy, adolescent health, violence prevention, and sports participation.

Global Action Network
953 Mission Street, Suite 111
San Francisco, CA 94103
Telephone: 415-512-1371; Fax: 415-512-1373
http://www.globalactionnetwork.org/

The Global Action Network is an online community designed to connect, educate, and empower young people working in the global population and reproductive health field. The network allows young people to connect to innovative peers and organizations around the world, as well as to discover opportunities for global training, fellowships, and funding.

Kinsey Institute
Morrison Hall 302
1165 East Third Street
Bloomington, IN 47405
Telephone: 812-855-7686; Fax: 812-855-8277
http://www.kinseyinstitute.org/about/site-index.html

The mission of the Kinsey Institute is to promote interdisciplinary research and scholarship in the fields of human sexuality, gender, and reproduction. The institute carries out this mission through the development of specialized collections of resources for scholars; programs of research and publication; interdisciplinary conferences and seminars; provision of information services to researchers; and graduate training.

National Education Association Health Information Network
1201 Sixteenth Street NW
Washington, DC 20036
Telephone: 202-822-7570
http://www.neahin.org/

The NEA Health Information Network (NEA HIN) recognizes that HIV/AIDS, sexually transmitted diseases, and unintended pregnancy are major public health concerns, and it has programs and publications to help school personnel address these issues in their roles as educators and as employees. NEA HIN provides members with publications that promote coordinated school health, effective models of HIV prevention education for the classroom, and accurate information on sexual health issues.

National PTA
330 North Wabash Avenue, Suite 2100
Chicago, IL 60611
Telephone: 312-670-6782; Fax: 312-670-6783
http://www.pta.org/aboutpta/index.asp

National PTA is a volunteer child advocacy organization supplying developmentally appropriate sexuality education materials. PTA is a not-for-profit association of parents, educators, students, and other citizens active in their schools and communities.

Plain Talk
10041 Sixth Avenue SW
Seattle, WA 98146
Telephone: 206-767-9244
http://www.aecf.org/publications/plaintalk/

Plain Talk is a group of community members working to improve positive and honest communication between parents and children, encourage youths to make healthy choices, and reduce teen pregnancy and sexually transmitted diseases. Plain Talk offers parents classes and resources to help them talk about sex and health with their children.

Sex Education Forum, National Children's Bureau
8 Wakley Street
London EC1V 7QE
Telephone: 020-7843-6052
http://www.ncb.org.uk/sef/contact.htm

The Sex Education Forum is located in the United Kingdom and offers a wide range of information on sex and relationships education (SRE). The forum maintains that good quality SRE is an entitlement for all children and young people. The forum works with forty-nine member organizations to achieve this goal. The organization works with teachers and health professionals across all settings, promoting good practice through a range of publications and fact sheets.

**Sexuality Information and Education Council
of the United States (SIECUS)**
1706 R Street NW
Washington, DC 20009
Telephone: 202-265-2405; Fax: 202-462-2340
http://www.siecus.org

The Sexuality Information and Education Council of the United States (SIECUS) is a national nonprofit organization incorporated in 1964. SIECUS develops, collects, and disseminates information; promotes comprehensive education about sexuality; and advocates for the right of individuals to make responsible sexual choices. Areas of focus include dating, gender issues, safer sex, same-sex relationships, and pregnancy prevention.

Society for the Scientific Study of Sexuality (SSSS)
P.O. Box 416
Allentown, PA 18105-0416
Telephone: 610-530-2483; Fax: 610-530-2485
http://www.sexscience.org

The Society for the Scientific Study of Sexuality (SSSS) is an international organization dedicated to the advancement of knowledge about sexuality. It is the oldest organization of professionals interested in the study of sexuality in the United States. SSSS is an interdisciplinary group of professionals who believe in the importance of the production of quality research and the clinical, educational, and social applications of research related to all aspects of sexuality.

8

Selected Print and Nonprint Resources

This chapter provides readers with print and nonprint resources on the topics of dating and sexuality. For the dual purpose of organization and convenience, the chapter is divided into three parts. Part I provides 130 recommended books and is organized according to the sequence of topics presented in chapter 2. Part II supplies the reader with a listing of 28 research and online journals, and Part III provides 30 recommended videotapes or DVDs. The listings in Parts II and III are arranged alphabetically. All of the print and nonprint resources contained in this chapter are rather recent (post-2000 publication or release dates), and a brief review accompanies each.

Part I: Books

Dating and Sexual Values

Damon, William. 2002. *Bringing in a New Era in Character Education.* Stanford, CA: Hoover Institution Press.

In this book, a noted contributor in the field of moral development explores the importance of character development. This practical and applied book explains how adults can pass core values down to the next generation—including values involving developing sexuality—in ways that will benefit their conduct and life goals.

Dobrin, Arthur. 2002. *Ethics for Everyone: How to Increase Your Moral Intelligence.* New York: Wiley.

This book sheds valuable light on how moral choices are made, as well as how to better understand and analyze ethical dilemmas. The author provides thoughtful answers and solutions to tough real-world questions and issues.

Gibbs, John C. 2003. *Moral Development and Reality: Beyond the Theories of Kohlberg and Hoffman.* Thousand Oaks, CA: Sage.

Gibbs offers a solid contribution to the existing sexuality literature with this thought-provoking analysis of moral growth and development. It is loaded with insight about where society has been in the area of moral development, where it is now, and the issues and topics that need future investigation.

Gurian, Michael. 2000. *The Good Son: Shaping the Moral Development of Our Boys and Young Men.* East Rutherford, NJ: Penguin.

A captivating account of what adults can do to help younger generations develop a solid moral foundation to guide sound decision making. Gurian supplies a wealth of information, from how to understand moral reasoning abilities to how to reduce the communication gap that often exists between the generations.

Hoffman, Martin L. 2002. *Empathy and Moral Development.* Port Chester, NY: Cambridge University Press.

Hoffman explores how empathy and moral development are interwoven. Among the topics included are compassion for others in physical, psychological, or economic distress; feelings of guilt over harming someone; feelings of anger at others who do harm; and feelings of injustice when others do not receive their due.

Koehler, Michael D. 2003. *Coaching Character at Home: Strategies for Raising Responsible Teens.* South Bend, IN: Ave Maria Press.

This book explores the negative influences in youngsters' lives that threaten to overwhelm them, and discusses how parents can help to counter them. Koehler describes the importance of sound values and character and the importance of teaching children and teens to do the "right thing." He offers lively discussion, helpful and entertaining pointers, sample dialogues, and personal stories and anecdotes.

Martin, Michael. 2000. *Everyday Morality: An Introduction to Applied Ethics.* Florence, KY: International Thomas.

This book is an introduction to the study of morality as it applies to practical moral needs. Moral character is explored in such dimensions as virtues, vices, attitudes, emotions, commitments, and personal relationships. The book contains many applied examples of moral decision making.

Medhus, Elisa. 2003. *Raising Children Who Think for Themselves.* Lavergne, TN: Fine Communications.

The author offers a new approach to parenting that seeks to help parents raise empathetic, self-confident, moral, and independent thinkers. Many applied examples are interspersed throughout the book.

Murphy, Madonna M. 2002. *Character Education in America's Blue Ribbon Schools: Best Practices for Meeting the Challenge.* Blue Ridge Summit, PA: Scarecrow.

Promoting responsible citizenship and sound character are important school functions. This book examines school policies, programs, and practices that can foster such traits as well as nurture self-worth, democratic values, ethical judgment, and self-discipline.

Ryan, Kevin, and Karen E. Bohlin. 2003. *Building Character in Schools: Practical Ways to Bring Moral Instruction to Life.* New York: Wiley.

Ryan and Bohlin detail the principles and strategies of effective character education and explain what schools must do to teach students the habits and dispositions that lead to responsible adulthood. The authors include a useful resource section with sample lessons, program guidelines, and a parents' list of ways to promote character in their children.

Timmons, Mark. 2002. *Conduct and Character: Readings in Moral Theory.* Florence, KY: International Thomas.

A comprehensive look at recent contributions to the study of moral theory and ethics. Essays are organized according to a specified moral theory and are preceded by an introductory chapter that provides a conceptual framework for studying ethics.

Media Impact on Dating and Sexuality

Brown, Jane D., ed. 2001. *Sexual Teens, Sexual Media*. Mahwah, NJ: Erlbaum.

This book explores the research that has been done on the media's sexual context and its impact on adolescents, and it synthesizes the major findings. The research considers not only physical sex acts, but also the role the media plays in the development of gender roles, sexual orientations, standards of beauty, and courtship and relationship norms.

Gauntlet, David. 2002. *Media, Gender, and Identity*. Florence, KY: Routledge.

An introduction to the relationship between media and gender, including an assortment of examples from film, television, and men's and women's magazines. In this book, Gauntlet provides a balanced account of the changing landscape of popular media and culture.

Gunter, Barrie. 2002. *Media Sex: What Are the Issues?* Mahwah, NJ: Erlbaum.

Gunter explores the prevalence and prominence of sex in the media, public opinion concerning that content, and the use of sex as a selling device. Among the topics covered are the effects sometimes attributed to exposure to media sex, including degradation of women, rising teen pregnancy rates, and sexual assault.

Heins, Marjorie. 2001. *Not in Front of the Children: Indecency, Censorship, and the Innocence of Youth*. Gordonsville, VA: Farrar, Straus, and Giroux.

A fascinating look at "indecency" laws and other restrictions aimed at protecting youth. Heins takes readers through history by exploring such developments as Plato's argument for rigid censorship, Victorian laws aimed at repressing libidinous thoughts, and today's battles over sex education in public schools and attempts to regulate the mass media.

Holtzman, Linda. 2000. *Media Messages: What Film, Television, and Popular Music Teach Us about Race, Class, Gender, and Sexual Orientation*. Armonk, NY: Sharpe.

An interesting look at the positive and negative influences that the media have on American culture. Of particular interest is the evolution of film, television, and pop music, including the significance of each in creating opinions and role models with regard to race, class, gender, and sexual orientation.

Jennings, Bryant, Dolf Zillmann, and Aletha C. Huston, eds. 2001. *Media Effects: Advances in Theory and Research* Mahwah, NJ: Erlbaum.

A collection of articles designed to explore the scientific, psychodynamic, and clinical perspectives on the media. This is not a book for the beach, but certainly one for the bookshelves of serious-minded readers.

LaRue, Jan. 2002. *Protecting Your Child in an X-Rated World*. Nashville, TN: Focus on the Family.

LaRue offers readers a detailed look at why pornography is a danger to families, and then examines the many sides to its pervasiveness. A particular emphasis is placed on developing practical responses to stop pornography, from how to keep it out of one's home to how to help the child who has already been exposed to pornography.

Patterson, Philip D. 2002. *Stay Tuned: What Every Parent Should Know about the Media*. Sevierville, TN: Covenant House.

The media's negative influences are the focus of this book, most notably the sex, violence, vulgarity, and shock value that often enter the household by way of the media. Patterson explores what parents need to know and what needs to be done to protect younger generations.

Petley, Julian. 2001. *The Media: The Impact on Our Lives*. Vancouver, BC: Raincoast.

An examination of a variety of Internet issues, including censorship versus freedom of information, various types of Internet crimes, and implications for future policy. The author also looks at the influence that newspapers, radio, television, film, and advertising have on public perceptions of the world.

Pomerance, Murray, ed. 2001. *Ladies and Gentlemen, Boys and Girls: Gender in Film at the End of the Twentieth Century*. Buffalo: State University of New York.

Examines gender roles in contemporary foreign and Hollywood films amidst today's changing social, political, cultural, and economic conditions. Among other topics, Pomerance explores how films have treated such topics as sexual orientation, female power, and male intellectuality.

Internet Romance and Sex

Bronson, Po, and Richard Dooling. 2001. *Men Seeking Women: Love and Sex On-Line*. New York: Random House.

This book will allow readers to discover some of the dynamics of Internet courtship and romance. The stories provided by the authors are interesting and engaging.

Cooper, Albert, ed. 2002. *Sex and the Internet*. Bristol, PA: Taylor and Francis.

A professional reference book on a topic of growing importance. A range of articles covers many research areas and seeks to address the disturbing questions raised by sex and the Internet, especially the impact on younger generations.

Fein, Ellen, and Sherry Schneider. 2002. *The Rules for Online Dating: Capturing the Heart of Mr. Right in Cyberspace*. New York: Simon and Schuster.

The authors of this book provide communication strategies designed to foster healthy dating relationships on the Internet. The book shows all women—regardless of age, status, or computer knowledge—how to use electronic communication to relate to men in a way that maintains self-esteem and leads to healthy coupling.

Grundner, Thomas, M. 2000. *The Skinner Box Effect: Sexual Addiction and Online Pornography*. Gordonville, VA: Universe.

Grundner explores how online pornography represents an addiction and embraces all the characteristics of any other kind of addiction: mood alteration, compulsion, dependency, the need for higher and more exotic "doses," and withdrawal symptoms when the person tries to stop. For those suffering from the problem, Grundner provides an assortment of intervention strategies and ideas.

Jenkins, Philip. 2001. *Beyond Tolerance: Child Pornography Online*. New York: New York University Press.

This book is a disturbing, thought-provoking analysis of the distribution of hard-core child pornography. The author covers such topics as attempts to regulate postings on the Internet, privacy and censorship issues, and the inadequacies of traditional law-enforcement techniques to control the international scope and sophistication of the Internet and its users.

Lane, Frederick S. 2001. *Obscene Profits: The Entrepreneurs of Pornography in Cyber Age*. Bristol, PA: Taylor and Francis.

Provides a sobering look at how the Internet, phone sex, and adult films and videos have become a multi-billion dollar industry. Describes the role of changing social standards, aggressive marketing, and economic benefits of new technology in the growth of an industry that includes some of the nation's largest companies and thousands of new entrepreneurs.

Maheu, Marlene M., and Rona B. Subotnik. *Infidelity on the Internet: Virtual Relationships and Real Betrayal*. Naperville, IL: Sourcebooks.

The authors describe how millions of people worldwide are actively engaging in online sexual activity, reveling in the freedom and undefined boundaries of finding relationships in a virtual world. This important book examines the questions raised by this new type of relationship and provides couples with the information they need to face the challenges that the Internet brings.

McBain, Michael A. 2002. *Internet Pornography: Awareness and Prevention*. Gordonville, VA: Universe.

A good reference source about the problems accompanying unmonitored computer use among younger generations. McBain offers parents and other concerned adults the strategies to protect minors from questionable material on the Internet.

Raymond, Ilene. 2001. *A Parent's Guide to the Internet*. Los Angeles, CA: Mars.

This book presents all the technical information a parent needs to effectively monitor children's Internet use and experience. The book also features advice on parenting issues with the Internet; an analysis of parental control features such as filters; and interviews with Internet experts, educators, and child and adolescent professionals.

Sullivan, Michael. 2002. *Safety Monitor: How to Protect Your Kids Online*. Chicago, IL: Bonus.

A hands-on, step-by-step practical instruction book for parents. Sullivan shares how parents can take an active role in protecting their children from exploitation, sexual predators, adults-only content, pornography, and other harmful content that comes with computer and Internet access.

Dating and Club Drugs

Abadinsky, Howard. 2000. *Drugs: An Introduction*. Lexington, KY: International Thomas.

One of the better reference books available on all types of drugs, including club drugs. The author provides a broad and thorough understanding of drug abuse, exploring its biological, psychological, and social impact as well as its history, the business of drugs, drug laws, and law enforcement's response to illegal drugs.

Gahlinger, Paul M. 2001. *Illegal Drugs: A Complete Guide to Their History, Chemistry, and Abuse*. Las Vegas, NV: Sagebrush.

An overview of illegal drugs, including the psychology of addiction and the biological effect of drugs on the brain. The author details all major drugs by discussing their history, typical users, chemical characteristics, long-term health problems, and overdose information. A valuable reference source for students, parents, and healthcare professionals.

Hammersley, Richard, and Jason Ditton. 2001. *Ecstasy and the Rise of the Chemical Generation*. Florence, KY: Routledge.

Covers a wide range of topics on Ecstasy, including how people begin using it, types of users, ways of using the drug, problems and risks, and reasons for quitting. The authors conclude that all of the long-term/negative effects of Ecstasy are not completely known, and they suggest directions for future research.

Holland, Judy. 2001. *Ecstasy: The Complete Guide*. Rochester, VT: Inner Traditions International.

A look at how Ecstasy works; its promise as a treatment for depression, post-traumatic stress disorder, chronic pain, and other illnesses; and how to minimize the risk of its illicit use. This authoritative source has value for parents or professionals wanting the most recent and accurate reports on this drug.

Kuhn, Cynthia, Jeremy Foster, and Leigh Heather Wilson. 2000. *Buzzed: The Straight Dope about the Most Used and Abused Drugs from Alcohol to Ecstasy*. New York: Norton.

The authors of this book debunk myths and provide the details about such drugs as hallucinogens, opiates, inhalants, stimulants, nicotine, and alcohol. An engaging writing style makes the latest scientific research concise and easy to understand.

Measham, Fiona, Howard Parker, and Judith Aldridge. 2000. *Dancing with Drugs*. New York: New York University Press.

In this book, the authors detail many aspects of drug activity including the sociocultural context in which it occurs, health effects, attitudes of the participants, and issues of safety and security. Specific chapters cover the importance of identity issues, "clubbing" activities, coping strategies, and policy recommendations.

Parker, James N., and Phillip M. Parker, eds. 2002. *The Official Patient's Sourcebook on Club Drug Dependence*. New York: Icon Health.

This valuable sourcebook has been created for those choosing to make education and Internet-based research a part of the drug treatment process. Although it gives information useful to doctors, caregivers, and other health professionals, it also tells readers where and how to look for information covering virtually all topics related to club drug dependence, from the essentials to the most advanced areas of research.

Robbins, Paul R. 2001. *Designer Drugs*. Springfield, NJ: Enslow.

A comprehensive account of the development and effects of such compounds as MPTP, Speed, Ice, and Ecstasy. Robbins also identifies those factors (e.g., heredity, psychological motivations, family, and society) that put today's youth at risk.

Weatherly, Myra S. 2000. *Ecstasy and Other Drug Dangers*. Springfield, NJ: Enslow.

Weatherly clearly presents the dangers of Ecstasy, Crystal Meth, Crank, and other designer drugs, discussing their effects and addictive nature and the treatment of their abuse. One of the better books on the contemporary drug scene.

Wilson, Richard W., and Cheryl Kolander. 2003. *Drug Abuse Prevention, 2nd Ed.* Sudbury, MA: Jones and Bartlett.

An excellent overview of drug abuse and the various intervention modes available. The authors offer a holistic approach to planning and implementing a drug abuse prevention program.

Date Rape

Crompton, Vicki, and Ellen Zelda Kessner. 2003. *Saving Beauty from the Beast: How to Protect Your Daughter from an Unhealthy Relationship*. Boston: Little, Brown.

The authors provide advice for parents who might be anxious over their daughters' choice of boyfriends. This book offers solid background on all kinds of abuse, including physical assault and emotional battering, in a straightforward and sensitive fashion.

Gosselin, Denise K. 2000. *Heavy Hands: An Introduction to the Crimes of Family Violence*. Dallas, TX: Pearson.

This book explores the causes, consequences, and prevalence of domestic violence and the positive law-enforcement response. In addition to date rape, the author examines sibling abuse, rape and incest, child and elder abuse and neglect, male battering, and lesbian and gay violence.

Jasinski, Jana L., and Linda M. Williams. 2000. *Partner Violence.* Thousand Oaks, CA: Sage.

This volume covers critical aspects of partner violence, including date rape, marital rape, the effects of partner violence on children, partner violence among same-sex couples, and partner violence in ethnic minority couples. The volume is up to date and is a resource essential for students, researchers, and practitioners in all fields concerning the family.

Lindquist, Scott. 2000. *The Date Rape Prevention Book: The Essential Guide for Girls and Women.* Naperville, IL: Sourcebooks.

Author Lindquist informs readers that a woman is five times more likely to be raped by someone she knows than by a stranger. Lindquist supplies what everyone needs to know about this widespread crime.

Lloyd, Sally A., and Beth C. Emery. 2001. *The Dark Side of Courtship: Physical and Sexual Aggression.* Thousand Oaks, CA: Sage.

The negative interactions that take place between dating and courting partners, most notably physical aggression and sexual exploitation, rest at the foundation of this book. It emphasizes the importance of understanding how power dynamics, verbal aggression, interaction patterns, issues of control, and relationship dynamics are integrally tied to physical and sexual aggression.

Loue, Sana. 2001. *Intimate Partner Violence: Societal, Medical, Legal, and Individual Responses.* Hingham, MA: Kluwer Academic.

This is an excellent book for students, clinicians, and researchers. The author pays particular attention to the varied responses to partner violence and how responses at one level influence those at others. She is convinced that diminishing such violence requires addressing it as both an individual and a community issue.

Murray, Jill. 2001. *But I Love Him: Protecting Your Teenage Daughter from Controlling, Abusive Dating Partners.* Scranton, PA: HarperCollins.

This book is valuable reading for both parents and teenagers. Murray identifies the types of behaviors and situations that are a precursor to an abusive relationship, and the changes that are needed to promote trust, open communication, and harmony.

Pledge, Deanna S. 2002. *When Something Feels Wrong: A Survival Guide about Abuse, for Young People.* Minneapolis, MN: Free Spirit.

A look at what abuse is all about, how to get help, and how to put an end to abuse that is occurring. Pledge supplies valuable advice on where the abused can turn for intervention, how to find help, and what to expect during the healing journey.

Raine, Nancy V. 2000. *After Silence: Rape and My Journey Back.* Westminster, MD: Crown.

Raine exposes the misconceptions and cruelties that surround this crime with depth and detail. She discusses the long-term psychological and physiological after-effects of rape, its tangled sexual confusions, the treatment of rape by the media and the legal and medical professions, and contemporary cultural views of victimhood.

Tattersall, Clare. 2000. *Date Rape Drugs.* New York: Rosen.

Tattersall describes cases of rape in which the attacker is an acquaintance and uses drugs to make the victim defenseless. She also examines date rape drugs, including Rohypnol, and details how to prevent such attacks.

Same-Sex Dating

Baker, Jean M. 2001. *How Homophobia Hurts Children: Nurturing Diversity at Home, at School, and in the Community.* Binghamton, NY: Haworth.

Baker seeks to dispel the myths and misconceptions that exist about gays and to promote accurate and positive images. The author stresses the notion of diversity and acceptance and the removal of intolerant and insensitive perceptions of gays.

Beeman, Paul, and Bruce Koff. 2000. *Something to Tell You: The Road Families Travel When a Child Is Gay.* New York: Columbia University Press.

The authors show how families can thrive and grow through the creation of more honest relationships when a son or daughter comes out. This book contains a diverse collection of family stories in the hope of helping to break down widespread prejudice and put an end to destructive cultural myths.

Bernstein, Robert A. 2000. *Straight Parents, Gay Children: Inspiring Families to Live Honestly and with Greater Understanding.* New York: Avalon.

The author, a former national vice president of Parents, Families, and Friends of Lesbians and Gays (PFLAG), shares his account of how he came to terms with his daughter's homosexuality. A very sensitive and interesting narrative.

Carrington, Christopher. 2002. *No Place Like Home: Relationships and Family Life among Lesbians and Gay Men.* Chicago, IL: University of Chicago Press.

Carrington describes the manner in which gay relationships begin and endure over time, with a particular emphasis on domestic life. He shares with readers the experiences of creating and maintaining a home, including routines and activities of the inhabitants.

Clunis, Merilee, and Dorsey Green. 2000. *Lesbian Couples: A Guide to Creating Healthy Relationships.* New York: Avalon.

The authors provide lesbian couples with tools to handle such issues as living arrangements, work, money, coming out, and conflict resolution. Additionally, this book addresses personal and community issues such as monogamy and open relationships, transgender identity, and bisexuality.

Fairchild, Betty, and Nancy Hayward. 2000. *Now That You Know: A Parent's Guide to Understanding Their Gay and Lesbian Children.* Orlando, FL: Harcourt.

Fairchild and Hayward assist parents in responding supportively to gay children with advice emphasizing acceptance and affirmation. Of particular strength are chapters dealing with HIV/AIDS, gays and religion, and the concept of gay/lesbian marriages.

Kiminsky, Neil. 2003. *Affirmative Gay Relationships: Key Steps in Finding a Life Partner.* Binghamton, NY: Haworth.

Kiminsky sheds light on the complexities of gay relationships, including dating challenges and relationship dynamics. He underscores the importance of trust and commitment to foster relationship security and comfort.

Mancilla, Michael, and Lisa Troshinsky. 2003. *Love in the Time of AIDS: The Gay Man's Guide to Sex, Dating, and Relationships.* New York: Guilford Press.

One of the better books available on gay relationships, including how they are formed and maintained. Excellent coverage of the risks posed by HIV/AIDS.

Nimmons, David. 2002. *Soul beneath the Skin: The Unseen Hearts and Habits of Gay Men.* Gordonsville, VA: St. Martin's.

This book expounds upon the positive dimensions of being gay and the rewarding features of gay relationships. The book promotes the human worth of gays and lesbians, and highlights their full human and social potential within society.

Rich, Jason. 2002. *Growing up Gay in America.* Portland, OR: Franklin Street.

A well-written and informative book on being gay in the United States. The book provides answers to common questions and offers positive, practical, and accurate advice on a wide range of topics and issues currently facing gays.

Savin-Williams, Ritch C. 2001. *"Mom, Dad—I'm Gay": How Families Negotiate Coming Out.* Washington, DC: American Psychological Association.

The author shares the results of an extensive study exploring the coming-out experience for 164 adolescents. Quotes from the subjects make for interesting reading, as do the suggestions aimed at helping families and their children negotiate healthy relationships.

Premarital Sex

Barber, Nigel. 2002. *The Science of Romance: Secrets of the Sexual Brain*. Amherst, NY: Prometheus.

Whether readers are interested in sexual behavior during adolescence or during any other facet of the life cycle, this book will have appeal. Barber discusses such topics as physical attractiveness and sex signals, dating competition and aggression, and cheating and fidelity.

Crane, Betsy, and Robert Heasley. 2002. *Sexual Lives: A Reader on the Theories and Realities of Human Sexualities*. New York: McGraw-Hill.

This book focuses on the theoretical and the personal stories of people's sexuality. Personal narratives encourage the reader to think about how sexuality itself is "constructed" as a result of norms, values, beliefs, and practices.

Crooks, Robert L., and Karla Baur. 2001. *Our Sexuality*. Monterey, CA: Wadsworth.

A very readable book on human sexuality, one that includes coverage of all major topics. Extension coverage is given to sexual health and maintaining a responsible and healthy sexual relationship.

Hyde, Janet S., and John DeLamater. 2002. *Understanding Human Sexuality*. New York: McGraw-Hill.

This book discusses many topics applicable to the study of adolescent premarital sexual relations: contraception, teenage pregnancy, sexually transmitted diseases, and abortion.

Pallone, Nathaniel J. 2002. *Love, Romance, and Sexual Interaction: Research Perspectives from Current Psychology*. New Brunswick, NJ: Transaction.

This book of readings contains articles from social scientists, who address themes relevant to how times have changed with regard to gender and relationships. Dating in the age of AIDS is one of the many topics offered.

Parrott, Les, and Leslie Parrott. 2002. *Relationships: An Open and*

Honest Guide to Making Bad Relationships Better and Good Relationships Great. Grand Rapids, MI: Zondervan.

Designed for college students, young adults, singles, and dating couples, this book teaches the basics of healthy relationships, including friendship, dating, and the sharing of sexual intimacy. The authors are therapists and award-winning writers specializing in the study of relationships across the lifespan.

Peacock, Judith. 2001. *Dating and Sex: Defining and Setting Boundaries.* Mankato, MN: Capstone.

Peacock provides readers with basic information and guidelines for making decisions about sexual relationships. Among the topics are abstinence, birth control, and sexually transmitted diseases.

Ponton, Lynn. 2002. *The Sex Lives of Teenagers: Revealing the Secret World of Adolescent Boys and Girls.* New York: Bargain.

This book explores adolescents' sexual behavior and addresses controversial topics such as pregnancy, abortion, masturbation, sexual orientation, Internet dating, sexual risk taking, and gender roles. The book also supplies coverage of HIV/AIDS and teenage drug use.

Strong, Bryan, Christine DeVault, Barbara Sayad, and William Yarber. 2001. *Human Sexuality: Diversity in Contemporary America.* New York: McGraw-Hill.

Adolescent sexuality is one of the many topics featured in this nonjudgmental introduction to human sexuality. The strength of this book is its integration of ethnic, cultural, gender, and sexual orientation differences and similarities.

Tolman, Deborah. 2002. *Dilemmas of Desire: Teenage Girls Talk about Sexuality.* Cambridge, MA: Harvard University Press.

An intimate portrait of how teenage girls experience, understand, and respond to their sexual feelings and of how society mediates, shapes, and distorts this experience. The book is filled with captivating interviews in which adolescent females talk candidly about their many emotions with regard to sexuality.

Birth Control

Avraham, Regina, and Sandra Thurman. 2000. *The Reproductive System*. Broomall, PA: Chelsea House.

Describes the male and female reproductive systems; discusses the disorders and diseases of each; and examines sexually transmitted diseases, family planning, and infertility, giving information on prevention, treatment, and available options.

Bullough, Vern L., James A. Brundage, and Lois Robin. 2001. *Encyclopedia of Birth Control*. Santa Barbara, CA: ABC-CLIO.

Recognized scholars in the field present a thorough and detailed analysis of contraceptives both at home and abroad. A readable, engaging writing style blends with important coverage of the legal, political, and moral issues attached to birth control.

Connell, Elizabeth B. 2001. *The Contraceptive Sourcebook*. New York: McGraw-Hill.

This sourcebook provides comprehensive coverage of each contraceptive method, including a clear and understandable description of its advantages and disadvantages. The author has crafted a straightforward and jargon-free guide to birth control options.

Glasier, Anna, and Ailsa Gebbie. 2000. *Handbook of Family Planning and Reproductive Healthcare*. Orlando, FL: Churchill Livingstone.

The authors categorize and describe all of the major contraceptives available to couples today. Also, emphasis is placed on reproductive health and well being, the latter including safer sex practices.

Keyzer, Amy M., ed. 2000. *Family Planning Sourcebook: Basic Information about Planning for Pregnancy and Contraception*. Detroit, MI: Omnigraphics.

This reference book includes information on family planning issues and contraceptive choices. Includes a detailed glossary and an annotated list of helpful organizations.

Mucciolo, Gary. 2001. *Everything You Need to Know about Birth Control*. New York: Rosen.

The author discusses the reproductive system and the various methods of birth control and how they work. This is a good reference book, one that is thorough and written in a clear and understandable style.

O'Leary, Ann., ed. 2002. *Beyond Condoms: Alternative Approaches to HIV Prevention.* Hingham, MA: Kluwer Academic.

The purpose of this book is to provide a variety of options for HIV prevention and to stimulate ideas for future improvement for these methods in order to reduce or stop the spread of HIV. This book has particular appeal to students, parents, health educators, and public health professionals.

Tone, Andrea. 2002. *Devices and Desires: A History of Contraceptives in America.* Gordonsville, VA: Hill and Wang.

Previous books on the history of birth control have been written through the eyes of physicians, lawyers, and political activists. However, Tone breaks new ground by showing what it was really like to produce, buy, and use contraceptives during a century of profound social and technological change.

Watkins, Elizabeth S. 2001. *On the Pill: A Social History of Oral Contraceptives.* Baltimore, MD: Johns Hopkins University Press.

A fascinating account of the Pill's cultural and medical history, including the scientific and ideological forces that led to its development; the parts women played in debates over its application; and the role of the media, medical profession, and pharmaceutical industry in deciding issues of its safety and meaning.

Weschler, Toni. 2001. *Taking Charge of Your Fertility: The Definitive Guide to Natural Birth Control, Pregnancy Achievement, and Reproductive Health.* Scranton, PA: HarperCollins.

One of the better resources available for such topics as fertility awareness, birth control, and reproductive health. Numerous tables and graphs are presented clearly and without confusing medical jargon.

Teenage Pregnancy

Alpern, Michele, and Marvin Rosen. 2002. *Teen Pregnancy.* Broomall, PA: Chelsea House.

This book, aimed at adolescent audiences, provides good information on teen pregnancy, including a comparison of birth control methods along with information on how they work, effectiveness, side effects, where to purchase them, costs, and STD protection.

Borkowski, John, Keri Weed, and Thomas L. Whitman. 2002. *Interwoven Lives: Adolescent Mothers and Their Children*. Mahwah, NJ: Erlbaum.

In this book, the authors focus their energies on the complex circumstances inherent in teenage mothering and the relationship that is forged between caregiver and child.

Carr, Alan. 2002. *Prevention: What Works with Children and Adolescents*. Bristol, PA: Taylor and Francis.

This book deals with prevention and proactive strategies to combat the problem of teenage pregnancy. In addition, attention is devoted to other problems within the adolescent subculture: physical and sexual abuse, bullying, alcohol use and drug abuse, STDs and HIV infection, post-traumatic adjustment problems, and adolescent suicide.

Cherry, Andrew L., Mary E. Dillon, and Douglas Rugh, eds. 2001. *Teenage Pregnancy: A Global View*. Westport, CT: Greenwood.

A look at some interesting cross-cultural comparisons of teenage pregnancy. Fifteen different countries are explored in detail to give a global perspective of teenage pregnancy and to challenge students to think about how the problem should be addressed.

Cothran, Helen. 2001. *Teenage Pregnancy and Parenting*. Farmington Hills, MI: Gale Group.

This book is divided into three sections that address the extent and severity of adolescent pregnancy, contributing factors, and prevention. Among the topics explored are the effects on society of long-term welfare dependency, links between early childbearing and poverty, widespread acceptance of premarital sex, cohabitation, single motherhood, and the efficacy of sex education programs.

Ewing, Ann B. 2002. *Daycare and Diplomas: Teen Mothers Who Stayed in School.* Minneapolis, MN: Fairview.

A look at Minnesota's South Vista Education Center Teenage Mothers Program. This organization provides teen mothers with the assets they need to stay in school, be effective parents, and succeed in life.

Gottfried, Theodore. 2001. *Teen Fathers Today.* Washington, DC: Twenty-First Century.

Gottfried explores the emotional and lifelong impact of pregnancy on male adolescents. His straightforward, honest voice combines with real-life teen interviews to underscore his points.

Heller, Tania. 2001. *Pregnant! What Can I Do? A Guide for Teenagers.* Jefferson, NC: McFarland.

The author offers advice for the pregnant teenager in getting help, making the best choices, and building a better future. It provides in-depth discussion of the three choices—adoption, parenting, and abortion—available to pregnant teenagers and presents interviews with those who chose each of these options.

Leadbeater, Bonnie J., and Niobe Way. 2001. *Growing up Fast: Transitions to Early Adulthood for Inner-City Adolescent Mothers.* Mahwah, NJ: Erlbaum.

A thought-provoking analysis of the life experiences of low-income teenage mothers. The authors illuminate the diverse pathways and resilience that the women exhibit in their struggles to improve their lives and those of their children, and discuss program and policy implications of their findings.

Merrick, Elizabeth. 2000. *Reconceiving Black Adolescent Pregnancy.* Scranton, PA: Westview.

Merrick's work focuses on childbearing and adolescent development among lower-income African American teenagers. Of particular interest are the individual stories and themes of the participants in this study.

Sexually Transmitted Diseases

Alcamo, Edward. 2003. *AIDS: The Biological Basis.* Sudbury, MA: Jones and Bartlett.

Alcamo provides readers with an abundance of valuable information related to HIV/AIDS. He presents the most current body of knowledge about HIV/AIDS in addition to material devoted to the social implications of the disease.

Leman, Evelyn. 2000. *Safer Sex: The New Morality.* Buena Park, CA: Morning Glory.

This book looks to promote safer sex to protect teens from early, unwanted pregnancy and sexually transmitted diseases. Topics covered include family values, the influence of the media, HIV/AIDS and STDs, contraception, abstinence, sex education, abortion, and religion.

Matthews, Dawn D., ed. 2001. *Sexually Transmitted Diseases SourceBook: Basic Consumer Health Information about Sexually Transmitted Diseases.* Detroit, MI: Omnigraphics.

Provides readable, up-to-date information about the symptoms, diagnoses, and treatments of sexually transmitted diseases. Also covered are such topics as condom use, vaccines, STD education, and issues related to youth and adolescents.

Meeker, Meg. 2002. *Epidemic: How Teen Sex Is Killing Our Kids.* Fairfax, VA: Eagle.

A comprehensive examination of the wave of sexually transmitted diseases that have increased in recent years. Meeker explains the different types of STDs that exist and what teenagers need to do to reduce their chances of becoming victims.

Miller, David, and John Green, eds. 2001. *Psychology of Sexual Health.* Williston, VT: Blackwell.

For those readers desiring a book emphasizing the psychology of sexual health, this book is one of the more successful ones on the market. Various articles focus on the importance of sexual health and well being and how to maintain it.

Morse, Stephen A., King K. Holmes, and Ronald C. Ballard. 2003. *Atlas of Sexually Transmitted Diseases and AIDS.* New York: Elsevier.

One of the better reference books available on all aspects of STDs. The book contains a separate chapter on HIV/AIDS, more than 200 illustrations, and a detailed bibliography.

Perloff, Richard M. 2001. *Persuading People to Have Safer Sex: Application of Social Science to the AIDS Crisis.* Mahwah, NJ: Erlbaum.

The author explains why people practice unsafe sex, suggests ways to use communication to promote safer sex attitudes, and discusses influences of AIDS prevention campaigns. This book is a valuable resource for introducing students to the role that theory and research play in health communication and psychology.

Stine, Gerald J. 2003. *AIDS Update: 2003.* Old Tappan, NJ: Prentice Hall.

A recognized authority in the field supplies a comprehensive, authoritative, and up-to-date book on HIV/AIDS. It presents the entire 22-year chronology of the AIDS pandemic in a reasonable, logical, and scientific manner that interweaves biological, clinical, social, and legal discoveries.

Thompson, Suzanne, and Stuart Oskamp. 2001. *Understanding and Preventing HIV Risk Behavior.* Thousand Oaks, CA: Sage.

An integrated examination of behavioral research aimed at reducing the transmission of HIV. The authors tackle the critical question of how to influence people to change high-risk behaviors, particularly in the areas of sexual activity and drug use.

Yancey, Diane. 2002. *STDs: What You Don't Know Can Hurt You.* Brookfield, CT: Milbrook.

A thorough volume that discusses all bacterial, viral, and parasitic diseases. Symptoms and medical descriptions are straightforward and easy to understand, and considerations for healthy lifestyle choices are offered.

Living Together

Booth, Alan, and Ann C. Crouter, eds. 2002. *Just Living Together: Implications of Cohabitation for Children, Families, and Social Policy*. Mahwah, NJ: Erlbaum.

Among the topics in this volume are the historical and cross-cultural foundations of cohabitation, the role of cohabitation on contemporary family structure, and cohabitation's long- and short-term impacts on the well being of children.

Garascia, Anthony. 2002. *Getting Married, Living Together: A Guide for Engaged Couples*. South Bend, IN: Ave Maria.

A down-to-earth look at the challenges facing soon-to-be-married couples in the new millennium. The book is filled with practical advice and guidance.

Gramlett, Matthew D. 2002. *Cohabitation, Marriage, Divorce, and Remarriage in the United States*. Washington, DC: U.S. Government Printing Office.

Demographic trends and population profiles are featured in this paperback. This publication is a good reference source for research projects.

Haman, Edward A. 2001. *How to Write Your Own Premarital Agreement*. Naperville, IL: Sourcebooks.

Haman offers assistance to couples in drafting their own premarital agreements. This book includes a state-by-state summary of inheritance and divorce laws, along with premarital agreement forms and instructions.

Ihara, Toni Lynne, Ralph Berkley Warner, and Frederick Hertz. 2002. *Living Together: A Legal Guide for Unmarried Couples*. Berkeley, CA: Nolo.

This book confronts the legal gray area of couples living together. Partner rights and responsibilities are discussed, as well as obligations, agreements, and authorizations.

Mason, Mary Ann, Arlene Skolnick, and Stephen D. Sugarman. 2003. *All Our Families: New Policies for a New Century*. New York: Oxford University Press.

A scholarly investigation on all varieties of family life, including cohabitation. The book draws from research in sociology, psychology, social work, law, and public policy.

Miller, Robin, and Sandra Lee Browning, eds. 2000. *With This Ring: Divorce, Intimacy, and Cohabitation from a Multicultural Perspective.* New York: Elsevier.

This book is a collection of research articles that seek to examine specific marital processes from the perspective of diverse cultures. In particular, it focuses on the diversity that exists in law and divorce, intimacy, and cohabitation/alternative marital forms.

Solot, Dorian, and Marshall Miller. 2002. *Unmarried to Each Other: The Essential Guide to Living Together and Staying Together.* New York: Avalon.

This book is based on more than 100 interviews of unmarried partners across the country. Solot and Miller have written a very informative reference for those couples considering cohabitation or already cohabiting.

Waite, Linda J., Elizabeth Thomson, Christine Bachrach, and Michelle Hindin, eds. 2000. *The Ties That Bind: Perspectives on Marriage and Cohabitation.* Hawthorne, NY: DeGruytr.

This book's contributors examine the factors influencing the formation, timing, and form of marriage and cohabitation as well as the dramatic changes in these institutions in recent decades. Various articles focus on trends in marriage and cohabitation; perspectives on how unions are formed; values, attitudes, and norms about marriage; and economics.

Wu, Zheng. 2000. *Cohabitation: An Alternative Form of Family Living.* New York: Oxford University Press.

This book supplies an extensive analysis of cohabitation from the points of view of sociology, demography, and economics. Topics include cohabitation trends, why people choose cohabitation, childbearing, and the breakup of relationships.

Teenage Marriages

Adams, Susan. 2000. *The Marital Compatibility Test.* Omaha, NE: Addicus.

The author believes that marital compatibility can be measured before the ceremony (or before moving in together) by completing the items and exercises contained in this book. This test asks questions to help predict a couple's chances of living together in harmony.

Corral, Jill, and Lisa Miya-Jervis, eds. 2001. *Young Wives' Tales: New Adventures in Love and Partnership.* New York: Avalon.

A collection of essays from young wives who share their feelings about navigating the waters of legalized long-term relationships. The essays are as enlightening as they are engaging, and they show the diversity that exists in perceptions of love and partnership.

Donaldson, Corey. 2001. *Don't You Dare Get Married until You Read This: The Book of Questions for Couples.* New York: Crown.

Donaldson's book is designed to encourage partners to discuss their feelings openly before they walk down the aisle. The questions posed—ranging from playful to provocative—are designed to get partners talking frankly and communicating effectively about important relationship issues and challenges.

Halfon, Neal, Mark Schuster, and Kathryn McLearn. 2002. *Child Rearing in America: The Conditions of Parents with Young Children.* Port Chester, NY: Cambridge University Press.

This book draws from economics, sociology, developmental psychology, pediatrics, and health policy in its analysis of young families with infants and toddlers. Topics include preparation for parenthood, how families spend time together, family routines and practices, and domestic stresses and strains.

Morgan, Elisa, and Carol Kuykendall. 2002. *Children Change a Marriage.* Grand Rapids, MI: Zondervan.

This book is designed to meet the needs of parents of young children, including the changes and challenges that accompany the new arrival. Emphasis is placed on regaining equilibrium in the midst of new chores and responsibilities.

Nissinen, Sheryl. 2000. *The Conscious Bride: Women Unveil Their True Feelings about Getting Hitched.* Oakland, CA: New Harbinger.

A frank look at a bride's inner life that provides advance guidance, warning, support, and understanding for women getting married. Interviews with a group of young brides succeed in painting a realistic picture of the challenges facing newlyweds.

Paul, Pamela. 2002. *The Starter Marriage and the Future of Matrimony.* New York: Random House.

Drawing on more than sixty interviews with couples, Paul looks at the hopes and motivations of couples marrying today and examines the conflict between the cultural conception of marriage and the society surrounding it.

Phillips, Robert. 2000. *How Can I Be Sure? Questions to Ask before You Get Married.* Eugene, OR: Harvest House.

Reflecting the marital concerns of today, this workbook asks those considering marriage to respond to insightful questions about everything from their communication patterns to their future dreams.

Piver, Susan. 2000. *The Hard Questions: 100 Essential Questions to Ask before You Say "I Do."* East Rutherford, NJ: Putnam.

This book poses thought-provoking questions that challenge and inspire couples to build a lasting, intimate relationship. Piver focuses her questions on the key areas of married life, such as home, money, work, sex, community and friends, family, and spirituality.

Stark, Marge. 2001. *What No One Tells the Bride.* East Rutherford, NJ: Fine.

Stark interviews fifty married women, who tell their stories about marriage, reveal marital truths, and offer supportive advice to readers. The book is insightful, humorous, and compassionate and contains guidance from marriage counselors, ministers, financial advisors, and sex therapists.

Dating and Sexuality Education

Baumeister, Roy F. 2002. *Human Sexuality: Meeting Your Basic Needs.* Dallas, TX: Pearson.

This book discusses all aspects of human sexuality—from sexual anatomy and sexually transmitted diseases to gender roles and sexual orientation. The major concepts discussed are neither oversimplified nor overly technical.

Blake, Simon. 2002. *Sex and Relationships Education.* Dallas, TX: Fulton.

Blake has developed this guide for teachers or leaders working with adolescents in the areas of sex and relationship education. This is a useful, hands-on approach to guiding the formation and maintenance of healthy and stable teenage dating relationships.

Campos, David. 2002. *Sex, Youth, and Sex Education: A Reference Handbook.* Santa Barbara, CA: ABC-CLIO.

An authoritative handbook that compiles information and topics relating to sex education, including such issues as sexual violence against youth, sexual orientation, and youth with disabilities. The book also contains lists of organizations, associations, government agencies, and publications.

Caron, Sandra L. 2002. *Sex Matters for College Students: Sex FAQ's in Human Sexuality.* Dallas, TX: Pearson.

This brief, easy-to-read, affordable paperback is designed specifically for today's young adults to answer basic sexual questions in a friendly, nonthreatening, age-appropriate way. Utilizes a question/answer format.

Hutcherson, Hilda. 2003. *What Your Mother Never Told You about S-E-X.* East Rutherford, NJ: Berkley.

This is a very readable and straightforward book on sex. Hutcherson answers the questions women are reluctant to ask their mothers, don't ask their doctors, but need to know to be in charge of their bodies and their sex lives.

Irvine, Janice M. 2002. *Talk about Sex: The Battles over Sex Education in the United States.* Los Angeles: University of California Press.

Irvine offers a history of the culture wars over sex education and also provides an important examination of the politics of sexual speech in the United States. This is a very insightful and informative contribution to the sex education literature.

Lickona, Thomas, William Boudrea, and Judy Likona. 2003. *Sex, Love, & You: Making the Right Decision (Updated and Revised Ed.)*. South Bend, IN: Ave Maria.

These recognized researchers seek to dispel the myths and misconceptions about sexuality transmitted by the media and to replace them with a clear understanding of love and intimate relationships.

Moran, Jeffrey P. 2002. *Teaching Sex: The Shaping of Adolescence in the 20th Century*. Cambridge, MA: Harvard University Press.

Moran takes readers on a fascinating ride through the sexual past of the United States, exposing the various myths and trends established by the nation's sex education efforts. Moran captures the essence of various historical eras, including the moral anxieties of a nation deciding how to best teach the facts of life to younger generations.

Roffman, Deborah M. 2001. *Sex and Sensibility: The Thinking Parent's Guide to Talking Sense about Sex*. Scranton, PA: Perseus.

Roffman emphasizes the practical steps parents can take and the simple conversations they can have that will help steer children toward healthy sexual development. One of the better how-to books on the market.

Woody, Jane DiVita. 2001. *How Can We Talk about That? Overcoming Personal Hangups So We Can Teach Kids the Right Stuff about Sex and Morality*. New York: Wiley.

A well-written, down-to-earth resource that can help adults talk with children openly and honestly about sex. The author supplies excellent advice on providing children with meaningful moral guidance.

Part II: Journals and Online Publications

There are a number of research journals in the behavioral and social sciences that feature research in the areas of dating and sexuality. The following are particularly useful. The URL of each journal's website is included, along with a brief description of each journal's scope and/or purpose.

Counseling Psychologist
http://www.sagepub.co.uk/journals/details/j0178.html

Showcases new or developing areas of practice and research on topics of immediate interest to therapists and others in the helping professions.

Cross-Cultural Research
http://www.sagepub.co.uk/journals/details/j0072.html

Offers peer-reviewed articles that describe cross-cultural and comparative studies in all human sciences.

Culture, Health, and Sexuality
http://www.tandf.co.uk/journals/tf/13691058.html

This journal is broad and multidisciplinary in focus, containing contemporary research that is empirical as well as applied.

Ethnic and Racial Studies
http://www.tandf.co.uk/journals/routledge/01419870.html

One of the leading international journals for the analysis of race, ethnicity, and nationalism throughout the world.

Family Planning Perspectives
http://www.jstor.org/journals/00147354.html

This journal's many subjects include contraceptive practices, fertility levels, adolescent pregnancy, abortion, sexually transmitted diseases, and reproductive health.

Family Process
http://www.familyprocess.org/

Publishes family therapy and research appealing to social workers, family therapists, nurses, psychologists, physicians, clergy, and rehabilitation specialists.

Family Relations
http://www.ncfr.com/

An applied scholarly journal that emphasizes relationships across the life cycle and research with implications for intervention, education, and public policy.

Gender and Society
http://www.sagepub.co.uk/journals/details/j0135.html

Emphasizing theory and research, this publication aims to advance the study of gender and feminist scholarship.

Guide to the Internet
http://www.ed.gov/pubs/parents/Internet/

The U.S. Department of Education's *Guide to the Internet* website offers basic information about how to use a computer to find information and to communicate with others. It tells users how to get started on the Internet as well as how and where to locate resources for both parents and children. A particular emphasis is placed on how families can avoid encountering Internet materials that are obscene, pornographic, violent, racist, or offensive in other ways.

International Family Planning Perspectives
http://uk.jstor.org/journals/01903187.html

An international journal that focuses its energies on sexual and reproductive health issues, particularly in Africa, Asia, and Latin America.

Journal of Adolescence
http://www.elsevier.com/locate/issn/0140–1971

Provides a forum for all who are concerned with the nature of adolescence, whether they are involved in teaching, research, guidance, counseling, treatment, or other services.

Journal of Adolescent Research
http://www.sagepub.co.uk/

Provides readers with information on the ways in which individuals aged 10–20 develop, behave, and are influenced by societal and cultural perspectives.

Journal of Child and Family Studies
http://kapis.wkap.nl/journalhome.htm/1062–1024

An international forum for topical issues pertaining to the mental well being of children, adolescents, and their families.

Journal of Counseling Psychology
http://www.apa.org/journals/cou.html

Features empirical research in counseling activities, career development, diversity, and professional issues in counseling psychology.

Journal of Family Violence
http://www.kluweronline.com/issn/0885–7482

Explores all forms of family violence, including spouse battering, date rape, child abuse, sexual abuse of children, incest, abuse of the elderly, and marital rape.

Journal of Gay and Lesbian Social Services
http://www.haworthpressinc.com/

Dedicated to the development of knowledge that meets the practical needs of lesbians, gays, and bisexuals in their social context.

Journal of Gender Studies
http://www.tandf.co.uk/journals/ carfax/09589236.html

An interdisciplinary journal that publishes articles relating to gender, including diversity of cultural backgrounds and differences in sexual orientation.

Journal of Homosexuality
http://www.haworthpressinc.com/

This journal gathers scholarly research on homosexuality, including sexual practices and gender roles and their cultural, historical, interpersonal, and modern social contexts.

Journal of Interpersonal Violence
http://www.sagepub.co.uk/journals/details/j0015.html

Focusing on both victims and perpetrators, this journal examines links between all types of interpersonal violence, exploring the similarities and differences that exist.

Journal of Lesbian Studies
http://www.haworthpressinc.com/

Promotes scholarship and commentary on lesbianism from an international and multicultural perspective.

Journal of Marriage and Family
http:/www.ncfr.com/authors/index.htm

Features original research and theory, research interpretation and reviews, critical discussion concerning all aspects of marriage and family, and book reviews.

Journal of Research on Adolescence
http://www.s-r-a.org/jra.html

Explores adolescence against the backdrop of cross-national, cross-cultural, gender, ethnic, and racial diversity.

Journal of Sex and Marital Therapy
http://www.tandf.co.uk/journals/pp/0092623X.html

Focuses on therapeutic techniques and outcomes, special clinical and medical problems, sexual functioning, and intimate relationships.

Journal of Social and Personal Relationships
http://www.sagepub.co.uk/journals/details/j0036.htm

This bimonthly journal explores such diverse topics as family systems, dating, divorce, remarriage, attachment, and the transitions of parenthood.

A Parent's Guide to Internet Safety
http://www.fbi.gov/publications/pguide/pguidee.htm

The Federal Bureau of Investigation's online publication *A Parent's Guide to Internet Safety* is a resource guide that explains how advances in computer and telecommunication technology allow children and teenagers to reach out to new sources of knowledge and cultural experiences, but also how the Internet leaves them vulnerable to exploitation and harm by computer sex offenders. This source helps parents to understand the complexities of online child exploitation and where to go for advice and assistance.

Sexual and Relationship Therapy
http://www.tandf.co.uk/journals/carfax/14681994.html

Focusing on sexual and marital functioning, this journal caters to academics and other researchers and to clinicians, therapists, and counselors.

Sexualities
http://www.sagepub.co.uk/journals/details/j0065.html

A journal covering the whole of the social sciences, cultural history, feminism, gender studies, cultural studies, and lesbian and gay studies.

Violence against Women
http://www.sagepub.co.uk/journals/details/j0062.html

Research within this journal focuses on sexual assault and coercion, date rape, domestic violence, incest, and sexual harassment.

Part III: Videos

The following is a listing of recommended educational videotapes on dating and sexuality. It is organized alphabetically, and each entry contains a brief description of the title, along with source information and addresses. The titles are mostly VHS format, although some are available in DVD and are noted accordingly.

American Adolescence
Length:	30 minutes
Date:	2001
Cost:	$89.95
Source:	Films for the Humanities and Sciences
	P.O. Box 2053
	Princeton, NJ 08543-2053
	Telephone: 800-257-5126; Fax: 609-275-3767
	http://www.films.com

This video explores the challenges and hurdles faced by today's teens and discusses how their hopes, fears, and expectations will shape American society.

Baby Love
Length:	57 minutes
Date:	2002
Cost:	$129.95

Source: Films for the Humanities and Sciences
            P.O. Box 2053
            Princeton, NJ 08543-2053
            Telephone: 800-257-5126; Fax: 609-275-3767
            http://www.films.com

As it explores teenage pregnancy, the video includes intervention and parenting programs. A panel of adolescent mothers speaks out on such topics as love, virginity, and parenting.

Being Gay: Coming Out in the 21st Century
Length: 20 minutes
Date: 2003
Cost: $89.95
Source: Films for the Humanities and Sciences
            P.O. Box 2053
            Princeton, NJ 08543-2053
            Telephone: 800-257-5126; Fax: 609-275-3767
            http://www.films.com

This video discusses the history of homosexuality in an open, sensitive, and candid fashion. It includes accounts and stories of people who have recently taken the step of coming out.

Club Drugs: From Rave to Grave
Length: 30 minutes
Date: 2000
Cost: $159.00
Source: NIMCO, Inc.
            102 Highway 81 North
            Calhoun, KY 42327-0009
            Telephone: 800-962-6662; Fax: 800-541-0007
            http://www.nimcoinc.com

The program discusses the drugs often used by young people attending all-night dance parties ("raves" or "trances") and the health and safety risks they pose. Also available in DVD.

Date Rape Backlash
Length: 60 minutes
Date: 2000
Cost: $195.00
Source: Media Education Foundation

26 Center Street
Northampton, MA 01060
Telephone: 800-897-0089; Fax: 800-659-6882
http://www.mediaed.org

The video gives an in-depth look at the epidemic nature of date rape, with a particular emphasis on the college dating scene.

Dating Bill of Rights
Length: 26 minutes
Date: 2001
Cost: $89.95
Source: Films for the Humanities and Sciences
P.O. Box 2053
Princeton, NJ 08543-2053
Telephone: 800-257-5126; Fax: 609-275-3767
http://www.films.com

As it presents basic guidelines on developing clear communications, this video avoids harmful stereotypes but also gives advice on preventing abusive situations.

Ecstasy: The Facts
Length: 21 minutes
Date: 2002
Cost: $139.95
Source: Human Relations Media
41 Kensico Drive
Mount Kisco, NY 10549
Telephone: 800-431-2050; Fax: 914-244-0485
http://www.hrmvideo.com

The program investigates the widespread use of the drug Ecstasy and the health risks it presents. It also reveals the troubling new danger of the Ecstasy lookalike drug, MDA. Available in DVD.

Electronic Storyteller
Length: 30 minutes
Date: 2000
Cost: $195.00
Source: Media Education Foundation
26 Center Street
Northampton, MA 01060

Telephone: 800-897-0089; Fax: 800-659-6882
http://www.mediaed.org

As a complement to the material in this book on the media and
dating, this video provides insight on corporate media and the
messages conveyed to the public.

Gay Couples: The Nature of Relationships
Length: 50 minutes
Date: 2000
Cost: $149.00
Source: Films for the Humanities and Sciences
            P.O. Box 2053
            Princeton, NJ 08543-2053
            Telephone: 800-257-5126; Fax: 609-275-3767
            http://www.films.com

As a case study approach that examines the lives of gay couples,
this video discusses the topics of communication, gender roles,
and intimacy.

He Said, She Said: Gender, Language, and Communication
Length: 50 minutes
Date: 2001
Cost: $349.00
Source: Insight Media
            2162 Broadway
            New York, NY 10024-0621
            Telephone: 800-233-9910; Fax: 212-799-5309
            http://www.insight-media.com

While taking an interesting look at the conversational styles of
men and women, noted linguistic expert Deborah Tannen examines such issues as directness and indirectness, the use of communication ritual, and the tendency to speak literally.

Healthy Relationships
Length: 35 minutes
Date: 2000
Cost: $89.95
Source: Films for the Humanities and Sciences
            P.O. Box 2053
            Princeton, NJ 08543-2053

Telephone: 800-257-5126; Fax: 609-275-3767
http://www.films.com

This video offers teenagers practical approaches to nurturing healthy behavior in themselves and those they date. A particular emphasis is placed on handling peer pressure and making sound choices.

How Can I Tell if I'm In Love?
Length: 50 minutes
Date: 2000
Cost: $29.95
Source: Teacher's Video Company
            P.O. Box 4455-03FS01
            Scottsdale, AZ 85261
            Telephone: 800-262-8837; Fax: 800-434-5638
            http://www.teachersvideo.com

Advice and suggestions are given by experts in such areas as dating, sexual intimacy, and commitment. The program includes interviews as well as audience participation.

Integrity
Length: 30 minutes
Date: 2000
Cost: $89.95
Source: Magna Systems
            500 Coventry Lane, Suite 200
            Crystal Lake, IL 60014
            Telephone: 800-203-7060; Fax: 815-459-4280
            http://www.magnasystemsvideos.com

This video complements the text material on sexual values in Chapter 2 of this book. It explores how integrity intertwines with character and how it is put to the test in everyday life.

Intimate Partner Violence
Length: 30 minutes
Date: 2003
Cost: $129.95
Source: Films for the Humanities and Sciences
            P.O. Box 2053
            Princeton, NJ 08543-2053

Telephone: 800-257-5126; Fax: 609-275-3767
http://www.films.com

This video is a profile of a community in Buffalo, New York, where the medical community, social and psychiatric services, police, and courts formed a coalition to reduce the incidence of partner abuse and to help the victims.

Love
Length: 52 minutes
Date: 2002
Cost: $129.00
Source: Films for the Humanities and Sciences
P.O. Box 2053
Princeton, NJ 08543-2053
Telephone: 800-257-5126; Fax: 609-275-3767
http://www.films.com

As a probing look at love, including the many rituals that surround it and the psychological dynamics that create it, this program features many of the leading experts on love and intimate relations. Also available in DVD.

Love, Love Me, Do: How Sex Differences Affect Relationships
Length: 51 minutes
Date: 2001
Cost: $239.95
Source: Films for the Humanities and Sciences
P.O. Box 2053
Princeton, NJ 08543-2053
Telephone: 800-257-5126; Fax: 609-275-3767
http://www.films.com

This video discusses the way sex-related differences in the brain may influence love, dating, marriage, reproduction, and parenthood.

Not One More Person: Avoiding HIV
Length: 30 minutes
Date: 2002
Cost: $139.00
Source: Human Relations Media
41 Kensico Drive

Mount Kisco, NY 10549
Telephone: 800-431-2050; Fax: 914-244-0485
http://www.hrmvideo.com

The program features six adolescents who recently tested positive for HIV. In their own words, viewers learn how they got infected and how it could have been avoided.

Pretty Colors: Inside America's Rave Culture
Length: 77 minutes
Date: 2002
Cost: $149.95
Source: Films for the Humanities and Sciences
P.O. Box 2053
Princeton, NJ 08543-2053
Telephone: 800-257-5126; Fax: 609-275-3767
http://www.films.com

An insider's look at the world of raves fueled by techno music and synthetic drugs such as Ecstasy and methamphetamines is the focus of this video. It is a gritty and impactful video.

Preventing Sexually Transmitted Infections
Length: 25 minutes
Date: 2002
Cost: $139.00
Source: Human Relations Media
41 Kensico Drive
Mount Kisco, NY 10549
Telephone: 800-431-2050; Fax: 914-244-0485
http://www.hrmvideo.com

This video provides students with all the facts about STDs, with a particular emphasis on prevention and the implementation of safer sex practices. The price includes an accompanying CD-ROM.

Red Flags: Avoiding Abusive Relationships
Length: 20 minutes
Date: 2002
Cost: $95.95
Source: Films for the Humanities and Sciences
P.O. Box 2053

Princeton, NJ 08543-2053
Telephone: 800-257-5126; Fax: 609-275-3767
http://www.films.com

Guidance is offered on situations involving sexual pressure, manipulation and obsessive behavior, abuse, and lying, and problem lifestyles.

Reviving Ophelia: Saving the Selves of Adolescent Girls
Length: 35 minutes
Date: 1999
Cost: $279.00
Source: Insight Media
             2162 Broadway
             New York, NY 10024-0621
             Telephone: 800-233-9910; Fax: 212-799-5309
             http://www.insight-media.com

Psychologist Mary Pipher examines the role of media and popular culture in shaping the identities of teenage girls. Special attention is given to relationships and sexuality.

Sex Talk
Length: 60 minutes
Date: 2000
Cost: $29.95
Source: Teacher's Video Company
             P. O. Box 4455-03FS01
             Scottsdale, AZ 85261
             Telephone: 800-262-8837; Fax: 800-434-5638
             http://www.teachersvideo.com

In straightforward discussion, this video gives information about such issues as contraception, STDs, unplanned pregnancies, promiscuity, abstinence, and love.

Sexual Stereotypes in the Media
Length: 37 minutes
Date: 2001
Cost: $149.95
Source: Films for the Humanities and Sciences
             P.O. Box 2053
             Princeton, NJ 08543-2053

Telephone: 800-257-5126; Fax: 609-275-3767
http://www.films.com

Sexual stereotypes as presented in film, television sitcoms, and advertisements are the focus of this video. It encourages viewers to examine the distortions that such sexual stereotypes create, as well as the ongoing sexual biases that nurture them.

Slippery Blisses

Length: 42 minutes
Date: 2001
Cost: $275.00
Source: University of California Extension, Center for Media
           and Independent Learning
           2000 Center Street, Fourth Floor
           Berkeley, CA 94704
           Telephone: 510-642-0460; Fax: 510-643-9271
           http://ucmedia.berkeley.edu/

This program is a fascinating, award-winning documentary on kissing. The video combines science, biology, sensuality, history, and provocative speculation about the magical quality of this activity.

Spin the Bottle: Sex, Lies, and Alcohol

Length: 45 minutes
Date: 2003
Cost: $275.00
Source: Media Education Foundation
           26 Center Street
           Northampton, MA 01060
           Telephone: 800-897-0089; Fax: 800-659-6882
           http://www.mediaed.org

In this video the problems associated with problem drinking and how the media distorts alcohol's properties to young people are explored. Implications for gender identities and sexual risk taking are also featured. Also available in DVD.

Teen Parents: Making It Work

Length: 20 minutes
Date: 2003
Cost: $89.95

Source: Films for the Humanities and Sciences
P.O. Box 2053
Princeton, NJ 08543-2053
Telephone: 800-257-5126; Fax: 609-275-3767
http://www.films.com

In this video the world of adolescent marriages and the challenges faced at home, in school, and in life are explored. Suggestions are given on how to achieve domestic stability, including involving reluctant teenage fathers in child care.

Teen Sexuality in a Culture of Confusion
Length: 40 minutes
Date: 2001
Cost: $99.00
Source: Media Education Foundation
26 Center Street
Northampton, MA 01060
Telephone: 800-897-0089; Fax: 800-659-6882
http://www.mediaed.org

This program investigates the forces influencing young people's decisions about sex, such as the media, peers, family, and religion. It features the lives of eight teens, who talk frankly about their lives and sexual feelings.

Tough Guise: Violence, Media, and the Crisis in Masculinity
Length: 82 minutes
Date: 2000
Cost: $275.00
Source: Media Education Foundation
26 Center Street
Northampton, MA 01060
Telephone: 800-897-0089; Fax: 800-659-6882
http://www.mediaed.org

The relationship between media images and the social construction of masculine identities are the focus of this video. It presents many implications for dating relationships. Also available in DVD.

Understanding Healthy Relationships and Sexuality
Length: 30 minutes

Date: 2001
Cost: $129.95
Source: Films for the Humanities and Sciences
             P.O. Box 2053
             Princeton, NJ 08543-2053
             Telephone: 800-257-5126; Fax: 609-275-3767
             http://www.films.com

Among the topics explored are the different types of intimate relationships that exist, factors that influence the formation and maintenance of relationships, and social and psychological perspectives on people as sexual beings.

Wedding Advice: Speak Now or Forever Hold Your Peace
Length: 60 minutes
Date: 2003
Cost: $275.00
Source: University of California Extension
             Center for Media and Independent Learning
             2000 Center Street, Fourth Floor
             Berkeley, CA 94704
             Telephone: 510-642-0460; Fax: 510-643-9271
             http://ucmedia.berkeley.edu/

This video utilizes an engaging blend of personal testimony, humor, and expert analysis to explore the challenges and hurdles of marriage. It also analyzes the social, economic, and political contexts of marriage.

Glossary

abstinence orientation   A sexual standard that advocates the avoidance of sexual intercourse.

anorexia nervosa   A type of self-imposed starvation common among teenage females.

baby boom   A sharp upswing in U.S. births between 1946 and 1964. Individuals born during this time are referred to as *baby boomers.*

bulimia   Gorging oneself with excessive amounts of food and then inducing vomiting or using excessive amounts of laxatives.

character education   Education for teenagers seeking to promote such positive standards of conduct as responsibility, respect, and caring.

club drugs   Dangerous chemical substances including Ecstasy, GHB, and Rohypnol.

coed sleepover   An overnight, mixed-gender gathering of teenagers in the home of one of the participants.

cohabitation   The status reserved for couples who are unmarried, living in the same household, and who share certain obligations equivalent to a spousal-type relationship.

coming out   An acceptance and disclosure of a person's sexual preference.

computer bulletin board   A virtual thumb-tack bulletin board that enables Internet participants to post messages, which in turn enable others to read and send responses.

cultural relativism   The belief that there is no universal standard of good or bad when evaluating cultures.

cultural role script   A preconception of how one should behave in a social setting in terms of appropriate goals, desirable qualities, and typical behaviors.

culture   Everything individuals do or have as members of society. Culture serves to identify, organize, and unify people who share a common way of life.

cyberspace romance   A romantic online relationship.

cyberspace stalking   The unwelcome, unwanted, and repeated harassment and surveillance by another person on the Internet.

date rape   Sexual assault that occurs in either serious and casual relationships.

date rape drugs   Drugs such as Liquid Ecstasy (Gamma-Hydroxybutyrate), which serve to immobilize a victim, impair his or her memory, and thus facilitate the act of rape.

dating   The social process by which two people meet, interact, and pair off as a couple.

DNA Lifeprint Card   A card designed to protect children from violence and other crimes. The child's DNA "fingerprint" is taken (the inside cheek is swabbed so that DNA can be obtained) and can be preserved for more than fifty years.

double standard orientation   A sexual standard asserting that sexual promiscuity, particularly premarital sexual relations, is acceptable for men but not for women.

e-mail   Electronic mail, a message from one person to another sent via telecommunications links between computers or terminals.

extrinsic values   Values derived from society's standards of right or wrong that are usually grounded in intellectual conviction.

fertility rate   The number of children that a woman can be expected to have over the course of her reproductive life.

Gamma-Hydroxybutyrate (GHB)   A club drug that is typically used in combination with alcohol and that is often the drug used by perpetrators in date rapes. GHB is a central nervous system depressant that can relax or sedate the body.

gender identity   The psychological awareness of being either male or female.

Generation X The generation of people born in the United States between 1965 and 1980.

hedonistic orientation See *permissiveness without affection orientation.*

instant message A form of electronic communication that allows users of the same service who are online at the same time to have immediate, one-on-one, private chats.

Internet A large computer network linking smaller computer networks worldwide.

intrinsic values Values that are internalized from personal experience and that represent those beliefs governing actual, everyday behavior.

Ketamine A club drug that is an injectable anesthetic capable of producing dream-like states and hallucinations.

lysergic acid diethylamide (LSD) A club drug classified as a hallucinogen that is capable of inducing abnormalities in sensory perceptions.

media Communication agents such as television, the Internet, radio, newspapers, and magazines.

methamphetamine A club drug that is classified as a toxic, addictive stimulant capable of affecting many areas of the central nervous system.

methylenedioxymethamphetamine (MDMA) A club drug, known popularly as Ecstasy, that is similar to the stimulant amphetamine and the hallucinogen mescaline. It can produce both stimulant and psychedelic effects.

Music Television (MTV) A cable television channel featuring a format of music videos.

nanotechnology A field of science seeking to control individual atoms and molecules to create computer chips and other devices that are thousands of times smaller than current technologies permit.

perceived invulnerability A distortion of reality that prompts people to think they are charmed or invincible, which in turn may prompt them to engage in risk-taking behaviors. Adolescents are prone to this type of thinking.

permissiveness with affection orientation A standard that views sexual activity as an extension of a meaningful intimate relationship.

permissiveness without affection orientation Also called the *hedonistic orientation,* a sexual standard emphasizing the importance of sexual pleasure and satisfaction rather than moral constraint.

procreational orientation A sexual standard emphasizing that coital activity is acceptable only within marriage for the purpose of having children.

rape An act of a sexual nature that is forced upon an unwilling victim or that an unwilling victim is forced to perform on someone else.

raves All night dance parties especially popular among teenagers and young adults. Also known as *trances.*

reality television A loosely scripted docudrama seeking to capture real-life situations for entertainment purposes.

Rohypnol A tasteless, odorless club drug that produces sedative and toxic effects, both of which are heightened with the concurrent use of alcohol.

sexual revolution Changes in thinking in the United States during the 1960s that focused on various aspects of human sexuality, including gender roles and sexual behavior.

sexual value orientation A belief about the purpose(s) of sexual activity and its place within an intimate relationship.

sexually transmitted disease (STD) A contagious infection that, for the most part, is passed on by intimate sexual contacts with others.

situational orientation A sexual standard suggesting that sexual decision making should take place in the context of the particular situation and between or among those involved.

stalking The unwelcome, malicious, and repeated harassment of another person, which causes that individual to feel emotional distress.

trances See *raves.*

value   What a person believes to be right or wrong, appropriate or inappropriate, or desirable and undesirable.

Victorianism   A period of time in the mid- to late 1800s characterized by heightened morality and a repressive attitude toward sexuality.

Index

Abortion
  access and unsafe procedures, 55
  among American teenagers, 3, 20, 53,
    60
  historical background, 9, 16–17,
    122–123, 125
  outside the U.S., 89–90, 93–94, 96,
    102–104, 108, 110, 164 (fig.)
  resources, 237
  RU 486, 90, 127
About Face, 177
Abstinence, 9, 55
  adolescents' reasons for choosing,
    54–55
  and the double standard orientation,
    29, **268**
  resources, 204–205, 238, 262
  use/effectiveness as birth control, 169
    (table)
  See also Abstinence orientation
Abstinence orientation
  defined, 29, **267**
  historical background, 6, 9, 15
  organizations and associations,
    204–205
  religious values and, 54–55, 101
  See also Abstinence
Acid, 43, 168–169 (table), **269**. *See also*
  Club drugs
Acquired immune deficiency syndrome.
  See HIV/AIDS
Action Coalition for Media Education,
  177
Action for Media Education, 177–178
Addiction
  to online activities, 38, 181, 229
  resources, 184–188, 230–232
  See also Club drugs; Drinking; Drugs
Addiction Resource Guide, 184–185
Administration for Children and
  Families, 215, 217
Adolescence Directory On-Line (website),
  204
Adolescent females
  AIDS infection rates, 19
  contraceptive use, 57 (*see also*
    Contraception)

first intercourse, 53, 55, 57, 94, 107,
    163 (fig.)
  and marriage, 67 (*see also* Teenage
    marriage)
  media portrayals of, 34 (*see also* Media)
  and online relationships, 39 (*see also*
    Internet: online relationships)
  premarital sex among, 16, 53–54 (*see*
    also Premarital sex)
  resources and organizations, 151,
    204–206, 219–220, 238, 262
  sexual and reproductive timeline,
    163 (fig.)
  STDs and HIV/AIDS among, 19, 61–63
    (*see also* HIV/AIDS; Sexually
    transmitted diseases)
  See also Adolescents; Body image; Date
    rape; Girls; Teenage mothers;
    Teenage pregnancy; Women
Adolescent males
  contraceptive use, 57 (*see also*
    Contraception)
  as fathers, 242, 264
  first intercourse, 53, 55, 57, 94, 107,
    163 (fig.)
  and marriage, 67 (*see also* Teenage
    marriage)
  media portrayals of, 34 (*see also* Media)
  premarital sex among, 16, 53–54 (*see*
    also Premarital sex)
  resources, 151–152, 264
  sexual aggression by, 45, 46 (*see also*
    Date rape; Sexual assault)
  sexual and reproductive timeline,
    163 (fig.)
  STDs and HIV/AIDS among, 63 [*see*
    also HIV/AIDS; Sexually transmitted
    diseases (STDs)]
  See also Adolescents; Men
Adolescent Reproductive Health, 195
Adolescents
  computer and Internet use, 19, 32,
    36–40, 162–163 (tables), 230 (*see also*
    Computers; Internet)
  demographics (in the U.S.), 1–2
  demographics (outside the U.S.), 94,
    101, 105

Adolescents, *continued*
  drug use statistics, 40–41 (*see also* Club
    drugs)
  employment, 68–69
  HIV/AIDS infection, 19, 61, 170 (table)
    (*see also* HIV/AIDS)
  marriage (*see* Teenage marriage)
  media use, 31–32, 35–36 (*see also*
    Media)
  mental/emotional development, 58,
    72–73, 135–136
  outside the U.S. (*see specific countries
    and geographic regions*)
  perceived invulnerability, 58, 72, 269
  pregnancy (*see* Teenage pregnancy)
  resources, 204, 252, 254–255 (*see also
    specific topics, such as* Dating and
    sexuality education)
  sexual activity (*see* Premarital sex)
  sexual and reproductive timeline,
    163 (fig.)
  stalking among, 49
  See also Adolescent females; Adolescent
    males
Adolescents after Divorce (Maccoby), 147
Advertising, 33
Advocates for Youth, 173–174
*Affirmative Gay Relationships: Key Steps
  in Finding a Life Partner* (Kiminsky),
  236
Africa
  abortion rate, 60
  adolescent poverty, 2
  AIDS infection rates, 170 (table)
  baby boomers, 13
  cohabitation, 64, 164 (fig.)
  North Africa, 100–102
  STDs and HIV/AIDS among, 63
  sub-Saharan Africa, 104–106, 111–112,
    126–127
African Americans
  teenage pregnancy and birth rate, 59,
    242
After Silence: Rape and My Journey Back
  (Raine), 234
Aggressive sexual behavior. *See* Date
  rape; Rape; Sexual assault; Violence
  and sexual violence
AIDS (acquired immune deficiency
  syndrome). *See* HIV/AIDS
AIDS Health Project, 208
AIDS: The Biological Basis (Alcamo), 243
AIDS Update: 2003 (Stine), 244
AIDSinfo, 208
Alan Guttmacher Institute, 52, 195–196
Alcoholic beverages. *See* Drinking
*All Our Families: New Policies for a New
  Century* (Mason, Skolnick, and
  Sugarman), 245–246
Alliance for a Media Literate America,
  178
Alliance for Children and Families, 188
Alliance for Young Families, 216

Alternatives to Marriage Project, 212
American Adolescence (video), 255
American Association for Marriage and
  Family Therapy, 216
American Association of Sexuality
  Educators, Counselors, and
  Therapists, 219
American Couples (Blumstein and
  Schwartz), 153
American Foundation for AIDS Research,
  209
American Social Health Association,
  208–209
American Society of Addiction Medicine,
  185
Annie E. Casey Foundation, 52, 196
Anorexia nervosa, 35, **267**. *See also* Eating
  disorders
Are You Hot? (television program), 33
Asian Americans
  AIDS infection rates, 170 (table)
  baby boomers, 13
  cohabitation, 64
  and domestic violence, 188
  population growth, 2
Asian Task Force against Domestic
  Violence, 188
*Ask the Children: The Breakthrough Study
  that Reveals How to Succeed at Work
  and Parenting* (Galinsky), 139
Association of Reproductive Health
  Professionals, 196
*Atlas of Sexually Transmitted Diseases and
  AIDS* (Morse, Holmes, and Ballard),
  244
Australia, 86–88
Automobiles, 7–9, 115, 117

Baby boomers, 13–17, 118, 121–122, 167
  (table), **267**
Baby Love (video), 255–256
Being Gay: Coming Out in the 21st Century
  (video), 256
Best Friends Foundation, 204–205
*Between Generations: The Six Stages of
  Parenthood* (Galinsky), 139
*Beyond Condoms: Alternative Approaches to
  HIV Prevention* (O'Leary), 240
Beyond Tolerance: Child Pornography Online
  (Jenkins), 229
Birth control. *See* Contraception
Birth control pill. *See* Oral contraceptives
Birth rates
  historical rates, 13, 117, 167 (table)
  teenage birth rates, 16, 58–59, 67
  See also Fertility rates
Blacks. *See* African Americans
Body. *See* Physical attractiveness
Body image, 4, 33–35, 74, 129–130
Bordo, Susan R., 129–130
Botswana, 106
Boys. *See* Adolescent males
Brazil, 53, 142

Bringing in a New Era in Character Education (Damon), 223
Brooks-Gunn, Jeanne, 130–131
Brown, Jane, 34
Building Character in Schools: Practical Ways to Bring Moral Instruction to Life (Ryan and Bohlin), 225
Bulimia, 35, **267**. *See also* Eating disorders
Burma, 2
But I Love Him: Protecting Your Teenage Daughter from Controlling, Abusive Dating Partners (Murray), 233–234
Buzzed: The Straight Dope about the Most Used and Abused Drugs from Alcohol to Ecstasy (Kuhn, Foster, and Wilson), 231

Calderone, Mary S., 131–132
California, 64, 171 (table)
Campaign for Our Children, 205
Canada, 59, 61, 164 (fig.)
Cars, 7–9, 115, 117
Casey, Annie E., 52. *See also* Annie E. Casey Foundation
Casual sex. *See* Hedonistic orientation; Sexual values
CDC (Centers for Disease Control and Prevention), 209, 210–211
Cell phones, 19, 25–26
Censorship, 115, 117, 119–121, 123, 125, 226–227
Center for AIDS Prevention Studies, 210
Center for Alcohol and Addiction Studies, 185
Center for Development and Population Activities, 200
Center for Education and Drug Abuse Research, 185
Center for Health and Gender Equity, 196–197
Center for Health Services, 210
Center for Media Education, 178
Center for Media Literacy, 178–179
Center for Online Addiction, 181
Center for the Advancement of Ethics and Character, 174
Center for the Fourth and Fifth Rs, 174–175
Center for the Improvement of Child Caring, 216
Center for the Study of Ethical Development, 175
Center for Treatment Research on Adolescent Drug Abuse, 186
Center on Adolescent Sexuality, Pregnancy, and Parenting, 205
Centers for Disease Control and Prevention (CDC), 209, 210–211
Character Counts/Josephson Institute, 174
Character education, 30, 69, **267**
    resources, 132–133, 174–177, 204–205, 223–226
    See also Sexual values: education and guidance

Character Education in America's Blue Ribbon Schools (Murphy), 225
Character Education Partnership, 175
Chat rooms, 19, 162 (table). *See also* Internet
Cherlin, Andrew J., 132
Child Rearing in America: The Conditions of Parents with Young Children (Halfon, Schuster, and McLearn), 247
Childnet International, 181–182
Children
    computer and Internet use, 36–37, 128, 162–163 (tables)
    divorce's effects on, 143, 155–156
    of gay/lesbian parents, 192
    HIV/AIDS infection, 170–171 (tables)
    male children preferred in India, 93
    missing/exploited children, 184
    sexual predators targeting children on the Internet, 34
    of teenage mothers, 60, 69
    of unmarried parents, 107
    See also Adolescent females; Adolescent males; Adolescents
Children Change a Marriage (Morgan and Kuykendall), 247
Children Now, 179
Children of Lesbians and Gays Everywhere, 192
Children's Partnership, 182
Children's Rights Council, 216–217
China, 3, 88–90
Chlamydia, 19, 61–62, 166 (fig.). *See also* Sexually transmitted diseases
Civil unions, 126–127
Clothing, 4, 7
Club drugs, 40–44, 74, **267**
    date rape drugs, 40, 42–43, 74, 234, **268** (*see also* Date rape)
    parental fears, 25
    popularity and availability, 40–41, 128
    resources and organizations, 184–188, 230–232, 256–257, 261
    signs and symptoms of use, 41–43, 44
    street terms and combinations, 168–169 (table)
    See also specific drugs, such as Ecstasy
Club Drugs: From Rave to Grave (video), 256
ClubDrugs.org, 186
Coaching Character at Home: Strategies for Raising Responsible Teens (Koehler), 224–225
Coalition for Marriage, Family, and Couples Education, 212
Coalition for Positive Sexuality, 175–176
Co-ed sleepovers, 18, **267**
Cohabitation (living together), 64–66, 75, **267**
    contemporary statistics (U.S.), 20, 64–65, 164 (fig.), 172 (table)
    historical background, 120, 124
    outside the U.S., 88, 91, 97, 101, 107, 109, 111

Cohabitation (living together), *continued*
  resources and organizations, 212–215,
    245–246
  same-sex partners, 164 (fig.), 172 (table)
*Cohabitation: An Alternative Form of Family
  Living* (Wu), 246
*Cohabitation, Marriage, Divorce, and
  Remarriage in the United States*
  (Gramlett), 245
Coles, Robert, 132–133
Coming out, 49–50, 74, 256, **267**
Communication
  and date rape, 47, 48
  parent-teen communication and sexual
    behaviors, 57–58, 70
  resources and organizations, 154–155,
    181, 213–214, 221, 257–258
  See also Cell phones; Internet; Media
Communitarian Network, 176
Community Anti-Drug Coalitions of
  America, 186–187
Computer bulletin boards, 34, 162 (table),
  267. *See also* Internet
Computer dating, 38–39. *See also* Internet:
  online relationships
Computers
  children's and teenagers' use of, 36–37,
    128
  historical background, 120, 123, 126
  See also Internet
Condoms, 9, 57
  effectiveness, 169 (table)
  and STD risk, 62, 169 (table)
  use outside the U.S., 87, 91, 100, 102,
    104, 110
  See also Contraception
Condoms, female, 126, 169 (table). *See
  also* Contraception
*Conduct and Character: Readings in Moral
  Theory* (Timmons), 225–226
*The Conscious Bride: Women Unveil Their
  True Feelings about Getting Hitched*
  (Nissinen), 248
Contraception, 55–58
  in China, 89
  historical background, 9, 16, 116, 118,
    120–121, 124–128, 152–153, 240
  in Indonesia, 94
  in Japan, 98
  in Latin America and the Caribbean, 100
  methods and effectiveness, 169 (table)
  in the Middle East and North Africa,
    102
  resources and organizations, 199–204,
    237–242, 251, 262
  in the Russian Federation, 103
  in sub-Saharan Africa, 106
  in Sweden, 108
  in the United Kingdom, 110
  use by adolescents worldwide, 87, 91,
    93, 106, 111
  use by American adolescents, 55–58, 87
  See also specific methods

Contraceptive patch, 127. *See also*
  Contraception
Contraceptive Research and
  Development Program, 200
The Contraceptive Sourcebook (Connell),
  239
Counseling Psychologist (journal/website), 251
Couple Communication, 213
Courtship
  historical background, 7, 9–11
  universal behaviors, 111
  See also Dating; *and specific countries and
    geographic regions*
Crank (methamphetamine), 40, 43,
  168–169 (table), **269**. *See also* Club
  drugs
Cross-Cultural Research (journal/website),
  251
*Crossing Paths: How Your Child's
  Adolescence Triggers Your Own Crisis*
  (Steinberg), 154
Cultural relativism, 3, **267**
Culture and dating/sexuality, 2–3, 67,
  251, **268**
  cultural role scripts, 6–10, **267–268**
  *See also specific countries, ethnic/racial
    groups, and geographic regions*
Culture, Health, and Sexuality
  (journal/website), 251
Cyberspace romance, 19, 38–39, 74,
  228–230, **268**. *See also* Internet: online
  relationships
Cyberspace stalking, 39–40, **268**

Dancing, 9, 116, 118, 120. *See also* Raves
Dancing with Drugs (Measham, Parker,
  and Aldridge), 231
*The Dark Side of Courtship: Physical and
  Sexual Aggression* (Lloyd and
  Emery), 233
Date rape, 45–49, 74, **268**
  date rape drugs, 40, 42–43, 46–47, 74,
    234, **268** (*see also* Club drugs; *and
    specific drugs*)
  prevention, 44, 48, 233
  resources and organizations, 188–191,
    232–234, 255–257, 259–260
Date Rape Backlash (video), 256–257
Date Rape Drugs (Tattersall), 234
The Date Rape Prevention Book (Lindquist),
  233
Dating, **268**
  age at first dating, 18
  cultural differences, 2–3
  functions, 1
  historical background, 4–17
  universal behaviors, 111
  See also Courtship; *and specific countries,
    issues, and topics*
*Dating and Sex: Defining and Setting
  Boundaries* (Peacock), 238
Dating and sexuality education, 69–73
  and contraceptive knowledge, 56

effective education, 70–73, 75
need for, 69–70
outside the U.S., 87, 90, 98, 103, 108–110
research and writing on, 131–133,
   141–143, 153
resources and organizations, 173–174,
   219–222, 248–250, 258–259, 262
SIECUS *Guidelines*, 142
See also Character education; Sexual
   values; *and specific topics, such as*
   HIV/AIDS
Dating Bill of Rights (video), 257
*Daycare and Diplomas: Teen Mothers Who
   Stayed in School* (Ewing), 242
DeLamater, John D., 133–134
Denmark, 97
Depo-Provera (contraceptive), 126, 169
   (table). *See also* Contraception
Designer Drugs (Robbins), 232
Development. *See* Adolescents:
   mental/emotional development;
   Psychological development theories
*Devices and Desires: A History of
   Contraceptives in America* (Tone), 240
Diaphragm (contraceptive device), 98,
   169 (table). *See also* Contraception
*Dilemmas of Desire: Teenage Girls Talk about
   Sexuality* (Tolman), 238
Dines, Gail, 18–19
Dittrich, Liz, 35
Division of Sexually Transmitted
   Diseases, 210–211
Divorce
   cohabitation and, 66
   historical statistics, 13, 124
   outside the U.S., 98, 107–108
   research and writing on, 132, 143, 147,
      155–156, 245–248
   and teenage marriage, 68, 75
   See also Marriage
DNA Lifeprint card, 26, **268**
Domestic violence. *See* Family violence
Donnerstein, Edward, 134
*Don't You Dare Get Married until You Read
   This: The Book of Questions for Couples*
   (Donaldson), 247
Double standard orientation, 29, 53–54, **268**
Drinking (alcohol)
   in the 1920s, 9, 116
   and date rape, 44, 46–47 (*see also* Date
      rape)
   resources and organizations, 184–188,
      231, 263 (*see also under* Addiction)
   and risk-taking behaviors, 58, 62, 72,
      263
Drug Abuse Prevention, 2nd Edition
   (Wilson and Kolander), 232
Drugs
   date rape drugs, 40, 42–43, 46–47, 74,
      234, **268**
   injecting drug users in Indonesia, 95
   resources and organizations, 184–188,
      230–232
   and risk-taking behaviors, 58, 72
   and STD risk/infection, 62, 95, 102,
      104, 171 (table)
   See also Club drugs; *and specific drugs*
Drugs: An Introduction (Abadinsky), 230

Eating disorders, 35, 129–130, 267
Ecstasy (MDMA; methylenedioxymeth-
   amphetamine), 40–42, 44, 128,
   168–169 (table), **269**
   resources, 231–232, 257
   See also Club drugs
Ecstasy and Other Drug Dangers
   (Weatherly), 232
*Ecstasy and the Rise of the Chemical
   Generation* (Hammersley and
   Ditton), 231
Ecstasy: The Complete Guide (Holland),
   231
Ecstasy: The Facts (video), 257
Education
   and employment, 69, 165 (fig.)
   and likelihood of
      marriage/cohabitation, 99
   resources, 182
   and teenage marriage, 68
   and teenage pregnancy/parenthood,
      60, 242
   See also Character education; Dating
      and sexuality education; *and under
      specific topics, such as* HIV/AIDS
Electronic Storyteller (video), 257–258
Elias, Maurice J., 134–135
Elimidate (television program), 33, 128
E-mail, 37, 127, 162–163 (tables), **268**. *See
   also* Internet
*Emotionally Intelligent Parenting: How to
   Raise a Self-Disciplined, Responsible,
   and Socially Skilled Child* (Elias,
   Tobias, and Freidlander), 135
Empathy and Moral Development
   (Hoffman), 224
Employment
   education and, 69, 165 (fig.)
   and teenage marriage, 68
   of women, 11, 118
Encyclopedia of Birth Control (Bullough,
   Brundage, and Robin), 239
Engender Health, 200–201
England. *See* United Kingdom
Epidemic: How Teen Sex is Killing Our Kids
   (Meeker), 243
Erikson, Erik H., 135–136, 140
*Ethics for Everyone: How to Increase Your
   Moral Intelligence* (Dobrin), 224
Ethics Resource Center, 176
Ethnic and Racial Studies
   (journal/website), 251
*Etiquette in Society, in Business, in Politics
   and at Home* (Post), 6–7, 116
ETR Associates, 197
*Everyday Morality: An Introduction to
   Applied Ethics* (Martin), 225

Everything You Need to Know about Birth Control (Mucciolo), 239–240
Extrinsic values, 28, **268**

Family and Home Network, 213
Family and Youth Services Bureau, 217
Family Care International, 201
Family Diversity Projects, 213
Family Education Network, 182–183
Family Health International, 201
Family Information Services, 214
Family life resources, 212–219, 251–255. *See also* Relationships
Family planning
  in China, 88–90
  in Ireland, 96
  in the Middle East and North Africa, 102
  organizations, associations, and agencies, 200–204
  in the Russian Federation, 103
  in the United Kingdom, 110
  See also Contraception; Family size; Fertility rates
Family Planning Perspectives (journal/website), 251
Family Planning Sourcebook: Basic Information about Planning for Pregnancy and Contraception (Keyzer), 239
Family Pride Coalition, 192
Family Process (journal/website), 251
Family Relations (journal/website), 251–252
Family size
  in China, 88–90
  extended families, 101
  historical background, 10
  in Indonesia, 94
  in Japan, 98
  in Sweden, 108
  See also Fertility rates
Family Support America, 218
Family Violence and Sexual Assault Institute, 188–189
Family Violence Prevention Fund, 189
Family violence, resources and organizations, 139–140, 188–190, 206, 232–233, 253, 259–260
FamilyCares, 217–218
Fatherhood (Parke), 150
Fathers
  resources, 150, 218, 219
  teenage fatherhood, 242, 264 (*see also* Teenage marriage; Teenage pregnancy)
  See also Men; Parents
Federal Bureau of Investigation (FBI), 40, 183
Fertility awareness (natural birth control), 169 (table), 240
Fertility rates, 161 (table), **268**

outside the U.S., 87–89, 91–94, 96, 98, 100–103, 105–106, 108–110
in the U.S., 8, 10, 13, 17, 161(table)
See also Birth rates
Films. *See* Movies
Florida, AIDS cases in, 171 (table)
For Better or for Worse: Divorce Reconsidered (Hetherington and Kelly), 143
France, 61, 65, 90–91, 164 (fig.)
Freud, Sigmund, 9, 12, 115, 136–137
Fromm, Erich, 137–138
Furstenberg, Frank F., Jr., 138
Fuzeon (anti-HIV drug), 128

Gabelnick, Henry, 56
Galinsky, Ellen, 138–139
Gamma-hydroxybutyrate (GHB), 40, 42, 168–169 (table), **268**. *See also* Club drugs
Gay and Lesbian Alliance against Defamation (GLAAD), 192–193
Gay and lesbian people, 49–52
  children of gays/lesbians, 192
  civil unions, 126–127
  cohabitation, 64, 164 (fig.), 172 (table)
  coming out, 49–50, 74, 256, **267**
  and HIV/AIDS transmission, 171 (table) (*see also* HIV/AIDS)
  homosexuality no longer considered mental illness, 123
  problems encountered by, 50–51
  relationship dynamics, 51–52, 74–75
  resources and organizations, 192–195, 234–236, 253–254, 256, 258
Gay Couples: The Nature of Relationships (video), 258
Gelles, Richard J., 139–140
Gender and Society (journal/website), 252
Gender identity, 50, **268**
Gender roles
  and adolescent sexual behavior, 54
  books on, 228
  in dating, 6, 7, 111
  in France, 91
  historical roles, 5–7, 8, 11
  in Latin America and the Caribbean, 99
  resources, 252, 253
  and sexual intimacy, 6
  in Sweden, 107
  in the United Kingdom, 109
Generation X (baby busters), 17–18, **269**
Genital herpes, 61, 166 (fig.)
Georgia, AIDS cases in, 171 (table)
GetNetWise, 183
Getting Married, Living Together: A Guide for Engaged Couples (Garascia), 245
GHB (gamma-hydroxybutyrate), 40, 42, 168–169 (table), **268**. *See also* Club drugs
Gilligan, Carol, 124, 140–141
Girls Incorporated, 205–206, 219–220
Girls, resources and organizations for,

151, 204–206, 219–220, 238. *See also*
    Adolescent females
Global Action Network, 220
Global Reproductive Health Forum,
    201–202
Go Ask Alice! (website), 197–198
Gonorrhea, 19, 61–63, 104, 166 (fig.)
*The Good Marriage: How and Why Love
    Lasts* (Wallerstein and Blakeslee), 156
*The Good Son: Shaping the Moral
    Development of Our Boys and Young
    Men* (Gurian), 224
Gordon, Sol, 141–142
*Growing Up Fast: Transitions to Early
    Adulthood for Inner-City Adolescent
    Mothers* (Leadbeater and Way), 242
Growing Up Gay in America (Rich), 236
Guide to the Internet (website), 252
*Guidelines for Comprehensive Sexuality
    Education, Kindergarten–12th Grade*
    (SIECUS), 142
Gunter, Barrie, 18–19, 226
Guttmacher, Alan, 52

Haffner, Debra W., 142–143
*Handbook of Family Planning and
    Reproductive Health* (Glasier and
    Gebbie), 239
*The Hard Questions: 100 Essential
    Questions to Ask before You Say "I Do"*
    (Piver), 248
*He Said, She Said: Gender, Language, and
    Communication* (Tannen video), 258
Health and Human Services, U.S.
    Department of, 215, 217
Healthy Relationships (video), 258–259
*Heavy Hands: An Introduction to the Crimes
    of Family Violence* (Gosselin), 232
Hedonistic orientation (permissiveness
    without affection), 15–16, 29–30, **269,**
    270
Hepatitis B virus (HBV), 61–62, 166 (fig.)
Herpes, genital, 61, 166 (fig.)
Hetherington, E. Mavis, 143
Hispanics
    abortion rate, 60
    baby boomers, 13
    cohabitation, 64, 164 (fig.)
    demographics, 2
    STDs and HIV/AIDS among, 63, 170
        (table)
    teenage birth rate, 59
    See also Latin America and the
        Caribbean
Historical background of dating and
    sexuality
    early 1900s, 4–8, 115–116
    1920s, 8–9, 116–117
    1930s, 10, 117–118
    1960s–1990s, 13–17, 120–127
    postwar years, 12–13, 118–120
    twenty-first century, 17–20, 127–128
    World War II, 10–11, 118

HIV/AIDS, 166 (fig.)
    among American teenagers, 19, 61,
        62
    education and prevention in the U.S.,
        142, 211–212, 220–221
    education and prevention outside the
        U.S., 90–91, 110–112, 142
    education and prevention resources,
        240, 243–244, 260–261
    exposure categories, 171 (table)
    fear of, 30
    historical background, 124, 125, 127
    research, 124, 128, 208, 209
    resources and organizations, 208–212,
        220–221, 235–236, 240, 243–244,
        260–261
    statistics (in the U.S.), 19, 61–63,
        125–126, 166 (fig.), 170–171 (tables)
    statistics (outside the U.S.), 61–63, 87,
        90–91, 93–96, 98, 100, 102, 104–105,
        110, 125–128
    in sub-Saharan Africa, 105, 106,
        111–112, 126, 127
    and teenage marriage, 67
    treatment, 127, 128, 166 (fig.)
    vaccine, 128
    in women, 19, 63, 128
Homeless teenagers, 63
Homework, 37, 162–163 (tables)
Homosexual people. *See* Gay and lesbian
    people
Households
    cohabitation statistics, 164 (fig.) ,172
        (table) (*see also* Cohabitation)
    by metropolitan residence status, 172
        (table)
    single-parent households, 2, 37, 107,
        165 (fig.), 172 (table) (*see also*
        Mothers, single)
    by type, 165 (fig.), 172 (table)
*How Can I Be Sure? Questions to Ask before
    You Get Married* (Phillips),
    248
How Can I Tell if I'm In Love? (video),
    59
*How Can We Talk about That? Overcoming
    Personal Hangups So We Can Teach
    Kids the Right Stuff about Sex and
    Morality* (Woody), 250
*How Homophobia Hurts Children:
    Nurturing Diversity at Home, at
    School, and in the Community* (Baker),
    234
*How to Write Your Own Premarital
    Agreement* (Haman), 245
Human immunodeficiency virus. *See*
    HIV/AIDS
Human papilloma virus (HPV), 61, 62,
    166 (fig.)
Human Rights Campaign, 193
Human Sexual Inadequacy (Masters and
    Johnson), 123, 148. *See also* Sexuality:
    Masters and Johnson's research

Human Sexual Response (Masters and Johnson), 15, 122, 148. *See also* Sexuality: Masters and Johnson's research
Human Sexuality: Diversity in Contemporary America (Strong, DeVault, Sayad, and Yarber), 238
Human Sexuality: Meeting Your Basic Needs (Baumeister), 248–249
Humez, Jean M., 18–19
Hyde, Janet S., 144, 237

I Only Say This because I Love You: Talking to Your Parents, Partner, Sibs and Kids When You're All Adults (Tannen), 155
Identification, 26
Identity formation
    and early marriage, 68
    Erikson's theory, 135–136
    gender identity, 50, **268**
    Maccoby's work, 147
    resources, 226
Illegal Drugs: A Complete Guide to Their History, Chemistry, and Abuse (Gahlinger), 230
Illinois, AIDS cases in, 171 (table)
In a Different Voice: Psychological Theory and Women's Development (Gilligan), 124. *See also* Gilligan, Carol
India, 92–93
Indonesia, 93–95
Industrialization, 4–5
Infidelity on the Internet: Virtual Relationships and Real Betrayal (Maheu and Subotnik), 229
Instant messaging, 37, **269**. *See also* Internet
Institute for 21st Century Relationships, 214
Institute for Gay and Lesbian Strategic Studies, 193
Institute for Reproductive Health, 202
Institute for Sex Research. *See* Kinsey Institute
Integrity (video), 259
International Family Planning Perspectives (journal/website), 252
Internet, 36
    addictiveness of online activities, 38, 181, 229
    chat rooms, 19, 162 (table)
    creation, 122
    e-mail and instant messaging, 37, 127, 162–163 (tables), **268**
    growth, 36, 124, 128
    information searches, 37, 162 (table)
    online relationships, 38–40, 74, 228–230
    parental monitoring, 19, 32, 230
    pornography on, 19, 33–34, 38, 74, 184, 229–230
    resources and organizations, 181–184, 227–228, 252, 254

safety, 34, 39–40, 181–183, 228–230, 252, 254
    sexual solicitation via, 34, 38
    stalking via, 39–40, 48–49
    teenagers' use of, 19, 32, 36–37, 162–163 (tables)
    See also Chat rooms; Cyberspace romance
Internet Pornography: Awareness and Prevention (McBain), 229–230
Interracial relationships, 64
Interwoven Lives: Adolescent Mothers and Their Children (Borkowski, Weed, and Whitman), 241
Intimate Partner Violence (video), 259–260
Intimate Partner Violence: Societal, Medical, Legal, and Individual Responses (Hingham), 233
Intimate Violence in Families (Gelles), 139
Intrauterine device (IUD), 16
    effectiveness, 169 (table)
    historical background, 9, 115, 123
    use outside the U.S., 89, 91, 98, 102
Invulnerability, perceived, 58, 72, **269**
Iran, 101, 102
Iraq, 102
Ireland, 95–97
Islamic culture, 100–102
Israel, 101, 102
IUD. *See* Intrauterine device

Japan, 3, 59, 97–98
Jefferson Center for Character Education, 176–177
Jewelry, 4, 7. *See also* Piercing
JHPIEGO Corporation, 202–203
Johnson, Virginia A., 15, 122, 123, 148–150
Journal of Adolescence (journal/website), 252
Journal of Adolescent Research (journal/website), 252
Journal of Child and Family Studies (journal/website), 252–253
Journal of Counseling Psychology (journal/website), 253
Journal of Family Violence (journal/website), 253
Journal of Gay and Lesbian Social Services (journal/website), 253
Journal of Gender Studies (journal/website), 253
Journal of Homosexuality (journal/website), 253
Journal of Interpersonal Violence (journal/website), 253
Journal of Lesbian Studies (journal/website), 253–254
Journal of Marriage and Family (journal/website), 254
Journal of Research on Adolescence (journal/website), 254
Journal of Sex and Marital Therapy (journal/website), 254

Journal of Social and Personal Relationships (journal/website), 254
Just Living Together: Implications of Cohabitation for Children, Families, and Social Policy (Booth and Crouter), 245

Kaiser Family Foundation, 179–180
Kazakhstan, 104
Kenya, 53
Ketamine, 40, 42, 168 (table), **269**
Kinsey, Alfred C., 12, 16, 118, 119, 144–145
Kinsey Institute, 118, 220
Kissing, 3, 263
Kohlberg, Lawrence, 140, 145–146
Kyrgyzstan, 104

Ladies and Gentlemen, Boys and Girls: Gender in Film at the End of the Twentieth Century (Pomerance), 228
Latin America and the Caribbean, 98–100
Latinos. *See* Hispanics
Lesbian Couples: A Guide to Creating Healthy Relationships (Clunis and Green), 235
Lesbians. *See* Gay and lesbian people
Lesotho, 106
Liberia, 105
LifePartners, 214
Living together. *See* Cohabitation; Marriage
Living Together: A Legal Guide for Unmarried Couples (Ihara, Warner, and Hertz), 245
Love. *See* Romantic love
Love (video), 260
Love in the Time of AIDS: The Gay Man's Guide to Sex, Dating, and Relationships (Mancilla and Troshinsky), 236
Love, Love Me, Do: How Sex Differences Affect Relationships (video), 260
Love, Romance, and Sexual Interaction: Research Perspectives from Current Psychology (Pallone), 237
Lysergic acid diethylamide (LSD; Acid), 43, 168–169 (table), **269**. *See also* Club drugs

Maccoby, Eleanor E., 146–147
Machismo concept, 99
The Male Body: A New Look at Men in Public and in Private (Bordo), 130
Mali, 105
Maltreatment and Adolescent Pregnancy and Parenting Program, 206
Manlove, Jennifer, 56
Manners between the sexes, 6–7
The Marital Compatibility Test (Adams), 247
Marriage
 age at first marriage (in the U.S.), 8, 10, 13, 17, 20, 163 (fig.), 166 (fig.)
 age at first marriage (outside the U.S.), 88–90, 92, 94, 96–97, 101, 103, 105, 107, 109, 111

arranged marriages, 3, 9, 89, 92, 97
cohabitation and, 65–66, 75 (*see also* Cohabitation)
contemporary statistics, 66–67, 166 (table)
cultural differences, 3 (*see also specific countries and geographic regions*)
duration linked to woman's age at first marriage, 68
eroding faith in, 66
gap between first intercourse and, 53, 94
historical background, 5–6, 8, 12–13, 117, 118, 166 (fig.)
polygyny, 101, 105
resources and organizations, 132, 156, 212–216, 245–248, 254, 265
and teenage pregnancy, 59, 67
See also Civil unions; Divorce; Relationships
Marriage, Divorce, and Remarriage (Cherlin), 132
Maryland, AIDS cases in, 171 (table)
Maslow, Abraham H., 147–148
Masters, William H., 15, 122, 123, 148–150
McDowell, Sophia, 38–39
MDMA. *See* Ecstasy
Media, **269**
 adolescent use of, 31–32, 35–36
 censorship, 115, 117, 119–121, 123, 125, 226–227
 impact on dating and sexuality, 15, 18–19, 31–36, 74, 111
 parental monitoring of adolescent use, 32, 35–36
 resources and organizations, 177–181, 183, 226–228, 257–258, 262–263, 264
 worldwide influence, 87, 91
 See also Internet; Movies; Music; Radio; Television
Media Effects: Advances in Theory and Research (Jennings, Bryant, Zillmann, and Houston), 227
Media, Gender, and Identity (Gauntlet), 226
Media Messages: What Film, Television, and Popular Music Teach Us about Race, Class, Gender, and Sexual Orientation (Holtzman), 227
Media Sex: What Are the Issues? (Gunter), 226
The Media: The Impact on Our Lives (Petley), 227–228
Media Watch, 180
Medical Institute for Sexual Health, 211
Men
 age at first marriage (in the U.S.), 8, 10, 13, 17, 20, 163 (fig.), 166 (fig.)
 age at first marriage (outside the U.S.), 88–90, 96–97, 101, 103, 105, 107, 109
 average age of husbands/cohabitants, 65
 double standard orientation, 29, 53–54, **268**

Men, *continued*
  in the early 1900s, 5, 6
  fatherhood, 150, 218, 219, 242, 264
  media portrayals of, 34, 264
  premarital sex among, 16, 53–54 (*see also* Premarital sex)
  sexual aggression by, 45–47 (*see also* Date rape; Sexual assault)
  sexual and reproductive timeline, 163 (fig.)
  as stalkers, 49 (*see also* Stalking)
  See also Adolescent males; Fathers; Gender roles; Marriage
Men Seeking Women: Love and Sex On-Line (Bronson and Dooling), 228
Men Stopping Rape, Inc., 189
Mentors, need for, 30–31
Methamphetamine (Speed; Crank), 40, 43, 168–169 (table), **269**. *See also* Club drugs
Methylenedioxymethamphetamine (MDMA). *See* Ecstasy
Middle East, 100–102
"Mom, Dad—I'm Gay": How Families Negotiate Coming Out (Savin-Williams), 236
Moral Development and Reality (Gibbs), 224
Morality
  books on, 124, 140–141, 223–226
  Kohlberg's theory of moral development, 146 (*see also* Kohlberg, Lawrence)
  See also Character education; Sexual values
Morality in Media (organization), 183
Mothers, single, 37, 107, 165 (fig.). *See also* Teenage mothers; Teenage pregnancy
Mothers' Voices, 211
Movies
  content codes/laws, 115, 117, 119, 123
  historical background, 115–119, 121, 122
  rating system, 122, 125
  resources, 227, 228
  See also Media
Multiple sexual partners, 62, 75. *See also* Permissiveness without affection orientation; Premarital sex
Music
  content warning labels, 125, 127
  historical background, 115–125, 127
  resources, 227
  rock music, 12, 14, 119–121, 122, 123
  See also Media
Muslims, 100–102

Nanotechnology, **269**
National Campaign to Prevent Teen Pregnancy, 198
National Center for Missing and Exploited Children, 184
National Center on Fathers and Families, 218

National Clearinghouse for Alcohol and Drug Information, 187
National Clearinghouse on Families and Youth, 218–219
National Coalition against Domestic Violence, 190
National Coalition for the Protection of Children and Families, 184
National Council on Alcoholism and Drug Dependence, 187
National Council on Child Abuse and Family Violence, 190
National Council on Family Relations, 214–215
National Education Association Health Information Network, 220–221
National Family Planning and Reproductive Health Association, 198
National Fatherhood Initiative, 219
National Gay and Lesbian Task Force, 193
National Institute on Drug Abuse, 186
National Institute on Media and the Family, 180
National Network for Youth, 206
National Organization on Adolescent Pregnancy, Parenting, and Prevention, 206–207
National Prevention Information Network, 209
National PTA (Parents and Teachers Association), 221
National Sexual Violence Resource Center, 190–191
National Teen Pregnancy Prevention Research Center, 207
National Youth Advocacy Coalition, 194
Native Americans, 13, 64, 164 (fig.), 170 (table)
Natural family planning (NFP; fertility awareness), 169 (table), 240
Network for Family Life Education, 198–199
New Jersey, AIDS cases in, 171 (table)
New York, AIDS cases in, 171 (table)
N-Generation, 17
Niger, 105–106
Nigeria, 104, 105, 142
No Place Like Home: Relationships and Family Life among Lesbians and Gay Men (Carrington), 235
Norplant (contraceptive), 125, 169 (table). *See also* Contraception
North Africa, 100–102
Northern Ireland. *See* United Kingdom
Not in Front of the Children: Indecency, Censorship, and the Innocence of Youth (Heins), 226–227
Not Me, Not Now, 207
Not One More Person: Avoiding HIV (video), 260–261

Now That You Know: A Parent's Guide to Understanding Their Gay and Lesbian Children (Fairchild and Hayward), 235

Obscene Profits: The Entrepreneurs of Pornography in Cyber Age (Lane), 229
Office of Population Research, 203
Office on Violence against Women, 191
The Official Patient's Sourcebook on Club Drug Dependence (Parker and Parker), 231–232
On the Pill: A Social History of Oral Contraceptives (Watkins), 240
Oral contraceptives
    effectiveness, 169 (table)
    historical background, 16, 120, 240
    use by American teenagers, 57
    use outside the U.S., 87, 91, 98, 100, 102, 110
    See also Contraception
Ortho Evra (contraceptive), 127. *See also* Contraception
Our Sexuality (Crooks and Baur), 237
OutYouth, 194

PAIRS Foundation, 215
Parents
    and adolescents' contraceptive knowledge/use, 57–58
    adult children living with, 96–98
    and cohabitation by offspring, 66
    and dating and sexuality education, 70
    and drug prevention, 44 (*see also* Club drugs)
    fatherhood research, 150
    gay/lesbian parents, 192
    and the Internet, 19, 32, 39–40, 230
    marriages arranged by (*see* Marriage: arranged marriages)
    parenting resources and organizations, 134–135, 139, 150, 154, 216–219, 247 (*see also specific topics, such as* Internet; Media)
Parents and Teachers Association (PTA), 221
Parents, Families, and Friends of Lesbians and Gays (PFLAG), 194
A Parent's Guide to Internet Safety (website), 254
A Parent's Guide to the Internet (Raymond), 230
Parke, Ross D., 150
Partner Violence (Jasinski and Williams), 233
Partnership for a Drug-Free America, 187–188
Peer pressure, 54, 109
Pennsylvania, 171 (table)
Perceived invulnerability, 58, 72, **269**
Permissiveness with affection orientation, 15, 16, 29, **270**
    and cohabitation, 65
    outside the U.S., 87, 91, 107, 109, 111

Permissiveness without affection (hedonistic) orientation, 15–16, 29–30, 269, **270**
Persuading People to Have Safer Sex: Application of Social Science to the AIDS Crisis (Perloff), 244
Physical attractiveness, 2, 3–4, 33–35, 74, 129–130, 237
Piercing, 2, 4
Pill, the. *See* Oral contraceptives
Pipher, Mary, 151, 262
Plain Talk, 221
Planned Parenthood Federation of America, 9, 116, 199
Polygyny, 101, 105
Population Action International, 203
Population Institute, 203–204
Population Reference Bureau, 204
Pornography
    historical background, 119
    on the Internet, 19, 33–34, 38, 74, 184, 229–230
    resources and organizations opposed to, 183, 184, 227, 229–230
    and the sexual revolution, 14, 15
Post, Emily, 6–7, 116
Poverty
    adolescents and, 2, 68–69
    and family planning, 106
    and STD infection risk, 63
    teenage mothers in, 60, 68
Pregnancy, 66, 106. *See also* Teenage pregnancy
Pregnant! What Can I Do? A Guide for Teenagers (Heller), 242
Premarital sex, 52–55
    adolescents' changing attitudes toward, 52, 54
    contemporary statistics (U.S.), 53, 75
    and the double standard orientation, 54 (*see also* Double standard orientation)
    first intercourse, 53, 55, 57, 94, 107, 163 (fig.)
    history, 6, 16, 145
    outside the U.S., 87, 96, 106–107, 109 (*see also specific countries and geographic regions*)
    peer pressure and, 54, 109
    and the permissiveness with affection orientation, 54 (*see also* Permissiveness with affection orientation)
    resources and organizations, 195–199, 237–238
    risks and consequences, 54–55, 111 (*see also* HIV/AIDS; Sexually transmitted diseases; Teenage pregnancy)
    and the sexual revolution, 15–16
    universal behaviors, 111
    See also Sexual values
Pretty Colors: Inside America's Rave Culture (video), 261

Preventing Sexually Transmitted Infections (video), 261
Prevention: What Works with Children and Adolescents (Carr), 241
Procreational orientation, 29, **270**
Project YES, 195
Promiscuity. *See* Permissiveness without affection orientation
Protecting Your Child in an X-Rated World (LaRue), 227
Psychological development theories
  Erikson's theory, 135–136
  Freud's theories, 136–137 (*see also* Freud, Sigmund)
  Steinberg's work, 154
Psychology of Sexual Health (Miller and Green), 243
PTA (Parents and Teachers Association), 221
Puberty, onset of, 53
Puerto Rico, AIDS cases in, 171 (table)

Radio, 116, 117, 118, 119
Raising a Child Responsibly in a Sexually Permissive World (Gordon and Gordon), 141–142
Raising Children Who Think for Themselves (Medhus), 225
Raising Emotionally Intelligent Teenagers (Elias, Tobias, and Friedlander), 135
Rape, 45, **270**
  resources and organizations, 188–191, 232–234, 255
  See also Date rape; Sexual assault
Raves, 40, 74, **270**. *See also* Club drugs
Real Boys Educational Programs, 151–152
Real Boys: Rescuing Our Sons from the Myths of Boyhood (Pollack), 152
Real Boys' Voices (Pollack), 152
Reality television, 33, 128, **270**
Reconceiving Black Adolescent Pregnancy (Merrick), 242
Red Flags: Avoiding Abusive Relationships (video), 261–262
Relationships
  duration and frequency in U.S. vs. other countries, 53
  factors for healthy relationships, 51
  homosexual relationships, 51–52, 74–75, 235–236, 258 (*see also* Gay and lesbian people)
  resources and organizations, 137–138, 212–215, 232–238, 245–246, 251–252, 254–255, 258–262, 264–265
  self-actualization theory and, 147–148
  See also Cohabitation; Dating and sexuality education; Family violence; Marriage; Teenage marriage
Relationships: An Open and Honest Guide to Making Bad Relationships Better and Good Relationships Great (Parrott and Parrott), 237–238

Religious values
  abstinence orientation and, 54–55, 101 (*see also* Abstinence orientation)
  family size and, 102
  Irish sexual behavior and, 95
Reproductive health
  organizations and associations, 195–202, 210–211
  resources (print, online, audiovisual), 239–240, 243–244, 252
  See also Contraception; HIV/AIDS; Sexually transmitted diseases (STDs); Teenage pregnancy
The Reproductive System (Avraham and Thurman), 239
Reviving Ophelia: Saving the Selves of Adolescent Girls (Pipher book/video), 151, 262
Risk-taking behaviors
  adolescent development and, 58, 72–73
  alcohol/drug use and, 72, 263 (*see also* Club drugs; Drinking; Drugs)
  and HIV/AIDS prevention, 244 (*see also* HIV/AIDS)
  parent-teen communication, 70
  and the sense of invulnerability, 58, 72, **269**
Rock music, 12, 119–121, 122, 123
Roe v. Wade, 16–17, 123. *See also* Abortion
Rohypnol, 40, 42–43, 47, 168–169 (table), **270**. *See also* Club drugs
Romantic love
  in the 1920s, 9
  Internet romance, 19, 38–39, 74, 228–230
  resources, 237, 260
  See also Cohabitation; Marriage; Relationships
Roofies. *See* Rohypnol
RU-486, 90, 127
The Rules for Online Dating: Capturing the Heart of Mr. Right in Cyberspace (Fein and Schneider), 228
Russian Federation, 59, 102–104, 142
Rwanda, 105

Safer Sex: The New Morality (Leman), 243
Safety
  date rape prevention, 44, 48, 233 (*see also* Date rape)
  Internet safety, 34, 39–40, 181–183, 228–230, 252, 254 (*see also* Internet)
  missing/exploited children, 184
  safer sex practices, 62, 87, 239–240, 243–244 (*see also* Contraception; HIV/AIDS)
  substance abuse (*see* Club drugs; Drinking; Drugs)
  See also Stalking
Safety Monitor: How to Protect Your Kids Online (Sullivan), 230

Same-sex dating, 49–52
  resources and organizations, 192–195,
    234–236
  See also Gay and lesbian people
Sanger, Margaret, 9, 12, 116, 121, 152–153
*Saving Beauty from the Beast: How to
    Protect Your Daughter from an
    Unhealthy Relationship* (Crompton
    and Kessner), 232
Schoolwork, Internet use for, 37, 162–163
  (tables)
Schwartz, Jill, 56
Schwartz, Pepper, 153
*The Science of Romance: Secrets of the Sexual
    Brain* (Barber), 237
Self-actualization theory, 147–148
Sex
  coercive sex (*see* Date rape; Sexual
    assault)
  first intercourse, 53, 57, 94, 107, 163 (fig.)
  and HIV/AIDS transmission, 171
    (table) (*see also* HIV/AIDS)
  Masters and Johnson's research, 15,
    122–123, 148–150
  media portrayals of, 74
  responsible sexual behavior, 34
  Victorian attitude toward, 5–6
  See also Contraception; Premarital sex;
    Sexuality
Sex and Relationships Education (Blake),
  249
*Sex and Sensibility: The Thinking Parent's
    Guide to Talking Sense about Sex*
    (Roffman), 250
Sex and the Internet (Cooper), 228
Sex education. *See* Dating and sexuality
  education
Sex Education Forum, National
  Children's Bureau, 221–222
*The Sex Lives of Teenagers: Revealing the
    Secret World of Adolescent Boys and
    Girls* (Ponton), 238
Sex, Love, & You: Making the Right Decision
    (Lickona, Boudrea, and Lickona),
    250
*Sex Matters for College Students: Sex FAQ's
    in Human Sexuality* (Caron), 249
Sex Talk (video), 262
*Sex, Youth, and Sex Education: A Reference
    Handbook* (Campos), 249
Sexual and Relationship Therapy (journal/
    website), 254–255
Sexual assault, 45, 49, 53, 74, 270
  resources and organizations, 188–191,
    232–234
  See also Date rape; Family violence
Sexual Behavior of the Human Female
    (Kinsey et al.), 119, 145
Sexual Behavior of the Human Male (Kinsey
    et al.), 118, 145
*Sexual Lives: A Reader on the Theories and
    Realities of Human Sexualities* (Crane
    and Heasley), 237

Sexual revolution, 13–17, 30, **270**
Sexual Stereotypes in the Media (video),
    262–263
Sexual Teens, Sexual Media (Brown),
    226
Sexual values, 27, **270**
  abstinence orientation, 6, 9, 15, 29,
    54–55, 101, 204–205, **267**
  and cohabitation, 65 (*see also*
    Cohabitation)
  double standard orientation, 29, 53–54,
    268
  education and guidance, 27–28, 30–31,
    35 (*see also* Character education;
    Dating and sexuality education)
  healthy values systems, 31
  importance of, 27
  intrinsic vs. extrinsic, 28, **268**
  outside the U.S., 87, 91, 92, 101, 107,
    109 (*see also specific countries and
    geographic regions*)
  permissiveness with affection
    orientation, 15–16, 29, 54, 65, 87, 91,
    107, 109, 111, **270**
  permissiveness without affection
    (hedonistic) orientation, 15–16,
    29–30, **269**, **270**
  procreational orientation, 29,
    270
  resources and organizations, 173–177,
    223–226, 259
  situational orientation, 29, **270**
Sexualities (journal/website), 255
Sexuality
  education (*see* Dating and sexuality
    education)
  Freud's theories, 136–137 (*see also*
    Freud, Sigmund)
  Kinsey's research, 12, 16, 144–145
  Masters and Johnson's research, 15,
    122–123, 148–150
  resources and organizations, 220, 222,
    237, 248–249, 251, 254–255, 264–265
  sexual and reproductive timeline,
    163 (fig.)
  sexual revolution, 13–17, 30, **270**
  Sorensen's research, 16
  Victorian sexual repression, 5–6
Sexuality Information and Education
  Council of the United States
  (SIECUS), 131, 142, 222
Sexually transmitted diseases (STDs)
  infection rates outside the U.S., 87,
    90–91, 93–96, 98, 100, 102–105, 110
  resources and organizations, 208–212,
    237, 238, 243–244, 260–261, 262
  risk of contracting, 19, 55, 61–63
  safer sex practices, 62, 87, 169 (table),
    261
  in the U.S., 3, 16, 19, 53, 61–63, 166
    (fig.)
  See also specific diseases, such as
    HIV/AIDS

Sexually Transmitted Diseases Sourcebook: Basic Consumer Health Information about Sexually Transmitted Diseases (Matthews), 243
SIECUS (Sexuality Information and Education Council of the United States), 131, 142, 222
Single-parent households, 2, 37, 107, 165 (fig.), 172 (table). *See also* Mothers, single; Teenage mothers
Situational orientation, 29, **270**
The Skinner Box Effect: Sexual Addiction and Online Pornography (Grundner), 229
Slippery Blisses (video), 263
Society for the Scientific Study of Sexuality, 222
Something to Tell You: The Road Families Travel When a Child is Gay (Beeman and Koff), 234–235
Sorensen, Robertson, 16
Soul beneath the Skin: The Unseen Hearts and Habits of Gay Men (Nimmons), 236
Speed (methamphetamine), 40, 43, 168–169 (table), **269**. *See also* Club drugs
Spermicides, 169 (table). *See also* Contraception
Spin the Bottle: Sex, Lies, and Alcohol (video), 263
Sponge, contraceptive, 124, 126, 128. *See also* Contraception
Stalking, 48–49, 74, **270**
  cyberspace stalking, 39–40, 48–49, **268**
  resources for victims, 189, 191
Stalking Resource Center, 191
The Starter Marriage and the Future of Matrimony (Paul), 248
Stay Tuned: What Every Parent Should Know about the Media (Patterson), 227
STDs. *See* Sexually transmitted diseases
STDs: What You Don't Know Can Hurt You (Yancey), 244
Steinberg, Laurence D., 153–154
Sterilization (female/male), 89, 100, 110, 169 (table)
Straight Parents, Gay Children: Inspiring Families to Live Honestly and with Greater Understanding (Bernstein), 235
Strasburger, Victor, 33–34
Sub-Saharan Africa, 104–106, 111–112, 126, 127
Sudan, 104, 105
Surviving the Breakup: How Children and Parents Cope with Divorce (Wallerstein), 155–156
Swaziland, 106
Sweden, 61, 65, 97, 106–108, 164 (fig.)
Syphilis, 61–63, 104, 166 (fig.)
Syria, 102

Taking Charge of Your Fertility: The Definitive Guide to Natural Birth Control, Pregnancy Achievement, and Reproductive Health (Wechsler), 240
Talk about Sex: The Battles over Sex Education in the United States (Irvine), 249–250
Tannen, Deborah, 125, 154–155, 258
Teaching Sex: The Shaping of Adolescence in the 20th Century (Moran), 250
Teen Fathers Today (Gottfried), 242
Teen Health and the Media (website), 180–181
Teen Parents: Making It Work (video), 263–264
Teen Pregnancy (Alpern and Rosen), 240–241
Teen Sexuality in a Culture of Confusion (video), 264
Teenage fathers, 242, 264. *See also* Teenage marriage; Teenage pregnancy
Teenage marriage, 66–69
  contributing factors, 67
  duration, 68
  outside the U.S., 87, 91, 94, 96–97, 103, 105, 107, 109, 111
  and pregnancy, 59, 67
  relationship dynamics, 68, 75
  resources and organizations, 215–219, 263–264
  U.S. statistics, 13, 17, 20, 67–68
Teenage mothers
  birth rates, 16, 58–59, 67
  as custodial parents, 19–20
  health risks, 60, 69
  outside the U.S., 92, 98
  poverty among, 60, 68
  resources and organizations, 205–206, 241–242, 255–256, 263–264
  See also Teenage pregnancy
Teenage pregnancy, 58–61
  birth rates, 16, 58–59, 67
  consequences for mother and child, 60, 69, 206
  and marriage, 59, 67
  outside the U.S., 92, 94, 96, 100, 103, 164 (fig.)
  prevention, 57, 204–208, 241–242 (*see also* Contraception; Dating and sexuality education)
  resources and organizations, 198, 199, 204–208, 237, 240–242, 255–256, 262
  risk of, 54–55, 57
  in the U.S., 3, 16, 19–20, 52–53, 57–61, 67, 124, 164 (fig.)
  See also Abortion; Teenage mothers
Teenage Pregnancy: A Global View (Cherry, Dillon, and Rugh), 241
Teenage Pregnancy and Parenting (Cothran), 241
Teenagers. *See* Adolescents
TeenAIDS, 211–212
Teenwire.com (website), 199

Television
  books on, 227
  historical background, 117–125, 126, 128
  reality television programs, 33, 128, **270**
  sexual content, 18–19, 32–33, 179–180
  See also Media
Temptation Island (television program), 33, 128
Ten Talks Parents Must Have With Their Children about Sex and Character (Schwartz and Cappello), 153
Texas, AIDS cases in, 171 (table)
Throwaway Dads (Parke), 150
The Ties That Bind: Perspectives on Marriage and Cohabitation (Waite, Thomson, Bachrach, and Hindin), 246
Today Contraceptive Sponge, 124, 126, 128. *See also* Contraception
Tough Guise: Violence, Media, and the Crisis in Masculinity (video), 264
Trances. *See* Raves
Transportation, 25. *See also* Cars
Turkey, 101
The Two Sexes: Growing Up Apart, Coming Together (Maccoby), 147

Unbearable Weight: Feminism, Western Culture, and the Body (Bordo), 129–130
Understanding and Preventing HIV Risk Behavior (Thompson and Oskamp), 244
Understanding Healthy Relationships and Sexuality (video), 264–265
Understanding Human Sexuality (Hyde and Delamater), 144, 237
Unemployment, 68, 117
The Unexpected Legacy of Divorce: A 25-Year Landmark Study (Wallerstein), 156
United Kingdom, 59, 61, 108–110, 164 (fig.)
University of Iowa Department of Communication Studies, 181
Unmarried to Each Other: The Essential Guide to Living Together and Staying Together (Solot and Miller), 246
Unmarried-partner households. *See* Cohabitation
Uzbekistan, 104

Vaginitis ("Trich"), 166 (fig.)
Values, **271**. *See also* Character education; Sexual values; Values education
Values education, 27–28, 74. *See also* Character education; Sexual values
Vermont, civil unions in, 126–127
Victorianism, 5–6, 8, **271**
Violence against Women (journal/website), 255
Violence and sexual violence
  against gays/lesbians, 50–51
  in the media, 32–33
  resources and organizations, 134, 253, 255, 264
  See also Family violence; Sexual assault
Virginity, 54. *See also* Abstinence orientation; Double standard orientation

Wallerstein, Judith S., 155–156
Wedding Advice: Speak Now or Forever Hold Your Peace (video), 265
What No One Tells the Bride (Stark), 248
What Your Mother Never Told You about S-E-X (Hutcherson), 249
When Something Feels Wrong: A Survival Guide about Abuse, for Young People (Pledge), 234
Whites, 2, 13, 164 (fig.), 170 (table)
Wilson, Barbara, 33–34
With This Ring: Divorce, Intimacy, and Cohabitation from a Multicultural Perspective (Miller and Browning), 246
Women
  age at first marriage (in the U.S.), 8, 10, 13, 17, 20, 163 (fig.), 166 (fig.)
  age at first marriage (outside the U.S.), 88–90, 92, 94, 96–97, 101, 103, 105, 107, 109
  AIDS infection rates, 19, 63, 128
  average age of wives/cohabitants, 65
  and the double standard orientation, 29, 53–54, **268**
  effects of the sexual revolution on, 14
  employment of, 11, 118
  female morality, works on, 124, 140–141
  media portrayals of, 34, 177 (*see also* Physical attractiveness)
  premarital sex among, 53–54 (*see also* Premarital sex)
  reproductive health resources (*see* Reproductive health)
  sexual and reproductive timeline, 163 (fig.)
  violence against (*see* Date rape; Family violence; Rape; Sexual assault; Violence and sexual violence)
  See also Adolescent females; Date rape; Gender roles; Marriage; Mothers

XTC. *See* Ecstasy

You and Your Adolescent: A Parent's Guide for Ages 10–20 (Steinberg), 154
You Just Don't Understand (Tannen), 125, 154
Young Wives' Tales: New Adventures in Love and Partnership (Corral and Miya-Jervis), 247

About the Author

Jeffrey S. Turner is a full professor of Human Development and Family Studies at Mitchell College. He has taught at the college level for over thirty years and has received numerous awards for distinguished teaching. He is the co-author of many college-level textbooks, which have sold over 185,000 copies and have been used in over 300 colleges and universities in the United States and abroad, including Japan, Poland, Australia, and the United Kingdom. Among his book titles are *Families in America* (ABC-CLIO), *Lifespan Development* (Holt, Rinehart, and Winston), *Relationships across the Lifespan* (Greenwood Press), *Marriage and Family: Traditions and Transitions* (Harcourt, Brace, and Jovanovich), *Contemporary Adulthood* (Holt, Rinehart, and Winston), *Exploring Child Behavior* (Brooks/Cole), *Basic Principles of Child Development* (W. B. Saunders), and *Human Sexuality* (Prentice-Hall). He is also the author of numerous articles and studies and has served as a book review critic for the magazine *Marriage and Family Living*.

earnest

45
50
100
42
45
90
81
89
92
___

50
48
100
42
48
100
81
89
100
___